QUESTIONS AND ANSWERS

This is the dramatic story of the rapid growth of chiropractic in just over half a century and its far-reaching effects on the health of millions throughout the world.

What is chiropractic and how can a doctor of chiropractic help you?

What is the domain of chiropractic? What methods are used? Can it care for herniated discs, asthma, high blood pressure, nervous and emotional disorders?

Why the long and bitter controversy between the medical and chiropractic professions?

What are the facts about the drugless and the drug approaches to health?

Read the thought-provoking answers to these and other questions about health and disease in YOUR HEALTH AND CHIROPRACTIC.

YOUR HEALTH
AND
CHIROPRACTIC

THORP McCLUSKY

Revised Edition by Julius Dintenfass, B.S., D.C.

PYRAMID BOOKS ▲ NEW YORK

This book is dedicated to the sick and to their hope;
and to the courageous men and women who never
cease the search for ways to make them well.

YOUR HEALTH AND CHIROPRACTIC

A PYRAMID BOOK
Published by arrangement with
Milestone Books, Inc.

PRINTING HISTORY
Milestone Books edition published June 1957
Pyramid revised edition published June 1962

Pyramid Books are published by Pyramid Publications, Inc.,
444 Madison Avenue, New York 22, New York, U.S.A

Contents

Foreword to Revised Edition   7

PART ONE—WHAT IS CHIROPRACTIC?

1. *You and Your Health*   13

2. *Chiropractic Comes of Age*   19

3. *A Revolution in the Healing Arts*   28

4. *A Visit to a Chiropractor*   40

5. *Man's Incredible Nervous System*   47

6. *Spinal Manipulation Through the Ages*   64

7. *The Growth of Chiropractic*   69

8. *X-ray and Chiropractic*   85

PART TWO—RESULTS ACHIEVED BY CHIROPRACTIC

9. *Seeking the Source of Good Health*   93

10. *Chiropractic in Head and Upper-Body Ills*   101

11. *Chiropractic in Visceral and Lower-Body
    Ills, Including "Low back" Conditions*   109

12. *Chiropractic in General Ills*   118

13. *Chiropractic in Children's Ailments*   124

14. *Chiropractic in Mental Ailments*   135

PART THREE—Your Health and the Inevitable
Advance of New Ideas

15. *Organized Medicine's Private War Against
    Chiropractic*   147

16. *Medicine's "Glass House"*   165

17. *Medical and Lay Opinions in Favor of
    Chiropractic*   179

18. *Medicine's About-Face*   192

19. *Today's Chiropractor*   203

20. *The Future—Can Chiropractic Help You?*   212

APPENDIX

A. *The Year the Chiropractic Act
   Was Passed In Each State and
   Province of Canada*   221

B. *Chiropractic Boards of Examiners
   in the United States and Canada*   222

C. *List and Classification of Insurance
   Companies Granting Recognition to
   the Chiropractic Profession*   233

D. *Chiropractic Colleges in the United
   States and Canada*   252

Foreword to the Revised Edition

Charles F. Kettering, president of the General Motors Research Corporation, once made a statement that might be used to sum up the story of chiropractic during the past sixty-seven years: "First they tell you you're wrong, and they can prove it. Then they tell you you're right, but it's not important. Then they tell you its important, but they've known it all these years."

The basic principles of chiropractic have won acceptance only after decades of vigorous struggle. Leaders and educators of the profession have devoted a large amount of time and energy to fighting for the very life of chiropractic against the attacks of entrenched authorities who have felt threatened by "something new."

Perhaps the expenditure of so much sweat and toil in combatting this bitter opposition explains why there are so few popular books on chiropractic. Fortunately, *Your Health and Chiropractic* by Thorp McClusky has helped to fill this gap.

No one, after reading this book, can fail to appreciate the foundation of chiropractic, its interesting history and development, its embattled fight to overcome prejudiced opposition, its therapeutic results, and what it means to the future of your life and health. In this book you will find the dramatic story of how chiropractic became the first profession to recognize the supremacy of the nervous system in health and disease. And you will learn how this principle produced the great practical revolution in the healing arts which brought better health to hundreds of thousands of men and women, some of whose actual cases and statistics are revealed in these pages.

Your Health and Chiropractic developed as a result of a lead article which Thorp McClusky wrote in *Man's Magazine* seven years ago. Reader interest was immediate and overwhelming. Nearly half a million reprints were distributed, arousing a national interest that was amazing. In response to such demand, Mr. McClusky decided to write a complete book on the subject, and he approached his task with an investigative passion and a desire for clinical verification that proved unique.

He gathered material, pro and con, from all over the country. He visited chiropractic offices and colleges, interviewed physicians and chiropractors alike. While not accepting every opinion set forth by every chiropractor, he nevertheless did not fail to cast a critical eye on the attacks leveled against the profession by those suspicious of its success.

A quarter of a century devoted to chiropractic as a practitioner, educator, and editor has convinced me that this profession is here to stay. Chiropractic is a profession with great potential. Further scientific research will establish the case for chiropractic in ever greater circles of opinion. Further research into the mysteries of our nervous system will give man greater and greater control over his body and his health. But in the following pages there is ample evidence of why chiropractic is now the second largest healing profession in the world.

The steadily increasing demand for information about chiropractic has created a need for a new edition of *Your Health and Chiropractic* in a paperback book for a larger audience. This second edition has been revised and enlarged with the addition of new, up-to-date material and the deletion of obsolete items.

In the revision and editing for this second edition I greatly appreciate the important assistance and counsel of the executive officers of the National Chiropractic Association, who supplied much new data. The recommendations and excellent co-operation of Dr. Ernest G. Napolitano, as the official representative of the International Chiropractors Association were invaluable. Mr. Ken Gingerich, Executive Director of the International Chiropractors Association was most helpful. I am grateful to all who have helped in making this revised edition a valuable source of information about chiropractic.

JULIUS DINTENFASS, B.S., D.C.

June, 1962
Brooklyn, New York

Part One

WHAT IS CHIROPRACTIC?

CHAPTER ONE

You and Your Health

"How are you?" "How have you been?" The usual greetings of almost anyone you meet. They reveal that health is a major preoccupation with almost everyone. It has been one of mankind's greatest concerns since man first learned to bathe his wounds in water and rub his painful big toe.

Other possessions seem of little importance when one does not have good health. You can't work well. You cannot enjoy recreation. You can't be happy in your relationships with other people.

You want success in your job or your business; you need the energy, enthusiasm, initiative, and ability that are important for success in this strenuous space age. You want happiness; you want the appreciation and respect of your loved ones. All this is possible when you have good health.

What, then, are the chances today to live a normally sick-free life? When you get sick, what are your chances of getting well quickly without an excessive loss of time and money?

Despite the many advances of science and medicine in dealing with problems of health and disease, there are startling facts which indicate that the state of health of our people is steadily worsening and that more and more persons are suffering from some disability that interferes with their normal daily activities.

In our space age, with its population explosion, the solving of health problems is becoming more complex. As soon as one major sickness is solved, there are new ones to take its place.

Public health, hygiene and better living conditions have cut down many of the old-time contagious diseases, only to be replaced by many new degenerative diseases caused by the stresses and strains of modern living.

The National Health Education Committee, in its most recent publication, *Facts on the Major Killing and Crippling Diseases Today—1961,* reveals that 17,000,000 people are disabled by mental and emotional disorders, 11,917,000 by heart and circulatory diseases and 11,250,000 people are disabled by arthritis and rheumatic diseases. These diseases are regarded as the three leading causes of disability today.

According to the National Health Survey, sickness was responsible for 599.1 million days lost from work by all persons of seventeen years and over during the year July, 1957 to June, 1958.

Translated into dollars and cents this indicates a tremendous cost to our nation. According to the National Health Education Committee: "Based on a minimum daily wage of $10.00 (eight hours at $1.25 per hour) these 599.1 million days of lost work represent a loss in earnings by those unable to work of almost six billion dollars. This is about two-thirds of the amount to be paid as interest on our entire public debt in 1960."

It is strange that in the United States, where scientific progress leads the world, the hospitals are crowded to capacity; a seriously-ill person frequently has to wait his turn for days and even weeks until a bed is available.

The shortage of medical doctors is acute, and is becoming more so.

We are donating astronomical sums for medical research in a multitude of fields, yet the hope of early conquest of numerous diseases remains small.

Medicine, which has accomplished wonders in many ways, is failing in numerous respects. More and more the public is coming to suspect that the "Man in White" is not so infallible after all; and that when a medical doctor says, "I have done everything for you that science can do and your condition is hopeless," he may be in error.

It may be that there are many approaches to healing which have been overlooked or ignored by the medical profession in its overwhelming concentration on drugs and surgery. If "the proof of the pudding is in the eating" is a sound criterion, there is certainly at least one such non-medical method of healing which has proven its value beyond any shadow of doubt. It is the fastest-growing healing art in the world, and its name is chiropractic (pronounced "ki-ro-prak'-tik").

Chiropractic did not come into existence until 1895; by coincidence, the same year that Roentgen discovered the X-ray. The Curies—Pierre and Marie—were on the verge of commencing their studies of the mysterious Becquerel rays, which led them in turn to the

15

discovery of radium. Sigmund Freud was still relatively unknown. Not until a decade later would Albert Einstein publish his paper on the *Electrodynamics of Moving Bodies,* which described his theory of relativity and which led ultimately to unleashing the mighty power of the atom.

In 1895, there was one chiropractor and one patient. Today, there are more than 25,000 chiropractors and thirty-five million chiropractic patients in the United States alone. This means that about one-sixth of our population has experienced the services of a chiropractor. The total of chiropractic patients within the boundaries of Continental United States is increasing at a rate of about two million a year.

In addition, chiropractic has spread far beyond our shores to include our territories and other possessions, and such nations as Great Britain and Ireland, Canada, Germany, France, Spain, Italy, the Scandinavian countries, Portugal, Belgium, Australia, New Zealand, the South American republics, India, Japan, Cuba, Greece, Switzerland, Union of South Africa, and Mexico. It is even practiced in the countries behind the "Iron Curtain."

How can we explain the phenomenal growth and demand for the services of the chiropractic profession during these last few decades?

Millions of sick people throughout the world have turned to chiropractic because it provides a cornerstone of our knowledge of the normal and abnormal functions of the human system. Chiropractic research has discovered an important correlation between errors in bodily mechanics and disease.

Chiropractic has played a great part in the scientific

16

revolution of modern times. Since the profession began sixty-five years ago, it has contributed new knowledge and new concepts to the modern study of health and disease.

Because of its great efficiency in making sick people well, there has been a temptation to take chiropractic for granted. But the success of chiropractic is due to the fact that it has made several important contributions to modern science. They are as follows:

1. *Anatomical disrelation can create functional disturbances in the body.* This great discovery blazed a trail for the need of the study of structural anatomy as relating to posture and body mechanics in the problems of health and disease.

2. *Disturbances of the nervous system are primary factors in the development of many disease conditions.* This concept was laid down in 1895, long before the scientific world was aware of the great significance of the nervous system in causing disease.

3. *Spinal subluxations (minor displacements of spinal bones) are a specific cause of nerve irritation or interference.* It was the chiropractic profession that centered attention upon the human spine and pelvis as a significant factor in disease processes.

4. *The viscero-spinal principle: nerve irritation at the spine may lead to a disturbance in the function of one or more internal organs of the body.* Today this concept has been confirmed by extensive neurological research.

These four principles make up the bedrock of chiropractic practice. They have resisted all kinds of vicious attacks for sixty-five years. Today they are vindicated by clinical results and scientific research throughout the world. Spearheaded by these principles, the growth and demand for this new healing art have helped chiropractic come of age.

CHAPTER TWO

Chiropractic Comes of Age

It is obvious that the merit of a healing art is reflected in the number of its patients. We have already noted that chiropractic is the fastest growing of all the healing arts, with more than thirty-five million patients in the United States and many millions more in other nations. Perhaps even more important, however, than the total number of chiropractic patients is the proportion of that total who can afford what they consider to be the best, or at least what they consider to be of unique merit.

In this group of chiropractic patients we find some of the world's most famous personalities, including the late John D. Rockefeller, Sr., who certainly could afford any sort of care he desired. During the final seven years of his long life, Mr. Rockefeller utilized the services of both medical doctors and a chiropractor, Dr. William Jensen. Following Mr. Rockefeller's death, one of his family sent Dr. Jensen two telegrams of appreciation for his services, the first referring to them as "splendid" and the second thanking the chiropractor "for past health for myself and many members of our household."

Among the long list of other chiropractic patients drawn from all walks of life have been presidents Coolidge and Eisenhower, for example, and such notables as Fred Allen, Belle Baker, Lucille Ball, Clara Bow, Attorney General Herbert Brownell, Eddie Cantor, Tony Canzoneri, Enrico Caruso, Broderick Crawford, Joan Crawford, Clarence Darrow, Glenn Ford, Mahatma Gandhi, Averell Harriman, Louis Hayward, August Heckscher, William Holden, Elbert Hubbard, Jack Dempsey, Mme. Chiang Kai-shek, Cullen Landis, Lillian Leitzel, Ted Lewis, Frederic March, Patsy Ruth Miller, Irene Rich, Eddie Rickenbacker, U. S. Senator Glen Taylor, and Rudy Vallee.

It is apparent that many of the above are persons to whom the glow of perfect health is, or was, an invaluable professional attribute. These people turned to chiropractic not only to restore health which may have deteriorated, but to preserve continuous good health.

Therefore, it is not surprising that many motion picture companies, to whom even a few hours lost during the shooting of a picture may cost many thousands of dollars, employ chiropractors to keep their stars and other personnel in top physical condition. In a recent production starring Robert Cummings, chiropractic care was credited with saving the film company some $120,000.

In sports employing high-salaried players chiropractors are often utilized to keep the players in tiptop shape and restore them to duty in the shortest possible time following illness or injury. In baseball, for example, many major and minor league teams employ chiropractors. They are not utilized as trainers.

According to Dr. Erle Painter, who for twelve years was staff chiropractor with the New York Yankees, their job is purely and simply to "secure and maintain in each player a correctly aligned spine and a supple musculature." How these, particularly the former, are essential to health and how the chiropractor achieves them will become apparent later.

Hard-boiled accident and health insurance companies are not inclined to pay out money in the settlement of claims unless they feel that valid service has been rendered. It is significant that over the years an increasing number of companies—including many of the giants—have accepted chiropractic as an effective healing art and pay the fees of chiropractors. The number of insurance companies in the United States today that recognize chiropractic on an equal basis with medicine is probably close to six hundred as this is written. The list of their names begins with Aetna Life Insurance Company and ends with United States Casualty Company.

Lloyd Sanders, president of Atlas Mutual Life Insurance Company, wrote recently, "I can prove beyond any doubt that for blood pressure and heart disease (the nation's number one killer) chiropractors are so far ahead that medical men will never catch up." He added that with chiropractic "one to two weeks is often the limit of claims, while medical doctors run for weeks and months and repeat claims after patients have been up for a few weeks . . . Medical doctors should have to take two years of the chiropractors' course. Then they would be better qualified to practice healing."

And in a follow-up letter Mr. Sanders added, "We

have always recommended chiropractors, especially for heart, hypertension, strains, sprains, lumbago, female diseases; also for many other diseases. We have had very satisfactory results when chiropractors were in attendance. In most cases the claims ran less time than those attended by medical doctors."

Executives in trade and industry are just as hard-boiled as insurance moguls. Yet, today, major industrial plants in at least twenty-one states employ chiropractors to look after the health of their employees. In Pennsylvania, Andrew J. Sordoni, former State Secretary of Commerce and president of Sordoni Enterprises, stated that chiropractic care returned disabled employees to their jobs "quicker and with less cost to the worker and the employer than any other mode of treatment." In Michigan, a large plant employing about three thousand workers sent its industrial accident cases to a chiropractor instead of a medical doctor. After a six months' trial of chiropractic, it found that the lost-time frequency rate had been cut from 60.25 to 20.88 per cent. In Kentucky, the huge Girdler Corporation switched from a medical doctor to a chiropractor as its health director after the company's president had utilized the services of a chiropractor personally for approximately fifteen years.

Many corporations that do not actually employ chiropractors give full recognition to chiropractic on the same basis as they do to medicine. Numerous associations and other groups have also at various times passed resolutions in favor of chiropractic. Among these are great industrial unions and the American Legion, Veterans of Foreign Wars, Disabled American Veterans, and Catholic War Veterans. In forty-three states workmen's compensation laws recognize chiropractic. The Railroad Retirement Board gives it full acceptance. Rulings by the U. S. Treasury now allow federal income tax deductions for chiropractic as well as for medical expenses.

In the Army—which has no chiropractic corps—chiropractors are assigned to the Medical Corps. The Selective Service Act recognized chiropractic as "necessary to the maintenance of the national health . . ." In forty-one states chiropractors are legally permitted to care for patients with infectious and contagious diseases; in thirty-six they are authorized to sign death certificates and other public health instruments; in seven they now have access to the facilities of tax-supported hospitals.

Considering the youthfulness of chiropractic and the above indications of its amazing acceptance by millions of patients and in many areas of business and government, chiropractic as a valid healing art appears to be established indeed.

However, the growth of chiropractic is only part of the story. To understand fully what it is accomplishing with multitudes of patients, it is necessary to go to the patients themselves. Their personal accounts of what chiropractic did for them—often after medicine had failed—are far more dramatic than any statistics.

Among the thousands of cases let us take a typical experience of a prominent man, Mr. James G. Blaine of New York City, president of the Midland Trust Company. He appeared some time ago before a public hearing of a Joint Legislative Committee of New York State to give his personal experience with chiropractic: "I have been a trustee of Roosevelt Hospital for a great many years and I have the highest regard and respect for the medical and surgical professions. I was brought up by a stepfather who, from 1901 to 1903, was the head of the College of Physicians and Surgeons, and at one time was head of Roosevelt Hospital; so that my lay knowledge of and respect for the medical world is second to nobody's. That is, the respect, not the knowledge.

"The reason I am here can best be told in the story of my wife. Ten years ago my wife was in a severe automobile accident and had her neck broken. I was told that it was one case in 10,000 that survived. She was put in a plaster cast and stayed in Nassau Hospital, Mineola, for many months. When she finally got out, she had several years of reasonable health, and then she commenced to suffer a great deal of pain in her head, in her shoulders, and in her arms, and that pain did not get any better with the years; it got worse. I endeavored to get at the root of this, in the medical world in this country, but we never found any cure for it.

"I took my wife abroad to a man in Paris, who was supposed to be a great expert on such ailments. He did his best. He sent her for a cure at Aix les Bains and still nothing happened, except that the pains got much worse.

"Along about 1939, a friend of mine said, 'There is a man in New York, a chiropractor, who I believe could help your wife,' and I said, 'I haven't any interest in chiropractic.' He said, 'Well, I think she would be helped by him.' I said, 'I will talk with Mrs. Blaine.' And I did, and she said no; she did not want anybody to touch her neck. Then just before Christmas in

1940, I was at luncheon downtown and I got a telephone message that my wife was desperately ill. I was terrified. I jumped in a taxi and had them call the doctor to meet me at the apartment. When we got there, we found Mrs. Blaine lying in bed. I thought she was dying. Her face was a sort of a green color, and she was partly unconscious. The doctor gave her adrenalin injections and she got around and stayed in bed from the week before Christmas until approximately the latter part of January. She still suffered these pains and she came to me one day and said, 'I would prefer to die rather than to continue with this terrible agony, particularly these pains in my head. The only other source I know of is this man your friend says is a chiropractor.' And I said that was all right by me, 'If that is what you want to do, that is what I want you to do.'

"So, I recall this very definitely, it was on Lincoln's Birthday. She went to this man first a few days before and had X rays taken by him. At that time he said, 'I don't know whether I can help you or not, but I think I can if you are willing to trust me.' And she told me that she liked the man and was perfectly willing to trust him.

"So on Lincoln's Birthday she had an appointment to get what the chiropractors call an adjustment. She did not want me to go with her, so I stayed home.

"She came back about two hours later and when she walked into the room there was an expression on her face that was highly indicative that something had happened, and had happened for the good. As she came into the room, she held her arm up and said, 'Here, for the first time in years I can read my wrist watch without glasses, and I just do not understand it, in two hours . . . and what is more the pressure in my head has been relieved.'

"Up to that time Mrs. Blaine could never be up for more than three or four hours in the day, because she got so tired and suffered so much she had to take to her bed and rest. Now, that was in 1941. She has never had any serious trouble since then. She has never been in any real, severe pain. Occasionally, she does not feel quite up to par and she gets an adjustment. When she gets that adjustment, she feels ten years younger, immediately. We are just like a lot of other people; we have been readjusting our lives. We have a farm up in northern Connecticut. She ran that farm last year without assistance—we could not find any help up there. She ran that farm all by herself. She not only did all the work around the house—cooking, making beds, and so forth, but she spent the rest of the day working in her vegetable garden and doing a lot of work unheard of two years ago or three years ago.

"Now, when I heard of this meeting today I told my wife that I felt such a great obligation to chiropractic because of what it had done for her, that I wanted the privilege and opportunity to show my appreciation by coming here and testifying in favor of chiropractic."

Thousands of chiropractic patients are firmly convinced, through personal experience, that chiropractic achieves a high percentage of outright cures or impressive degrees of improvement. They assert that the period of convalescence under chiropractic is shorter than under medical care. Finally, they stress that chiropractic usually costs far less than medical treatment. Some medical doctors like to observe that, of all persons, the patient knows least of all what is the matter with him or what is good for him. But from a common sense point of view, it would seem that the patient at least knows how he feels and whether he is getting better or worse. If the patient's own feelings are any criterion of the validity of a healing art, then chiropractic is a highly—often dramatically—successful method of curing the sick and keeping the healthy well.

CHAPTER THREE

A Revolution in the Healing Arts

Chiropractic is something new under the sun, and to this day only about one out of every eight Americans has actually gone to a chiropractor. Perhaps the simplest method of getting some first-hand knowledge about chiropractic is to describe its rapid development since its start in 1895, pay a visit to a chiropractor of today, and then describe in detail what chiropractic is and does. From this it will become apparent that chiropractic, while it may appear at first to be an extremely simple healing art, is actually a very involved and precise science.

Long after the Civil War, practitioners gained medical knowledge by serving a term of apprenticeship with some local M.D. Many gained knowledge of medicine while sweeping out offices, cleaning the M.D.'s stalls, currying his horses, or driving the M.D. around the countryside on his house calls.

In most academic institutions in these years, attendance was required for a limited time. Only in rare instances was the period longer than one year. It was not until the 1880's that laws were written stating that licensees in medicine must have graduated from a recognized medical college before obtaining admission to practice in a state. Many early medical doctors were of the itinerant type who traveled from town to town and peddled cure-alls or allegedly superior Indian herb cures. Some noted surgeons of the past were graduates of terms of a shorter duration than one year. One well-known surgeon actually attended a medical institution for the brief term of six months.

Back in 1895, Daniel David Palmer of Davenport, Iowa, was fifty years old and well recognized as an unusual man of parts. Born in 1845 in the little Ontario town of Port Perry, he had become interested in healing the sick while still a young man, and had emigrated to the United States where he practiced several of the numerous methods of healing then in vogue.

D. D. Palmer was an omnivorous reader and a diligent investigator of everything available that dealt with healing. He felt that far too many attempts to heal were conducted on a "by-guess-and-by-gosh" basis. If they appeared to work, well and good; if they didn't, try something else.

Palmer felt that the healing arts up to this time were characterized by a singular unwillingness to search for a basic, underlying cause of disease. He set down his impressions in a penetrating analysis:

"In the dim ages of the past when man lived in rude huts and rocky caves, even up to the present time, he resorted to charms, necromancy, and witchcraft for the relief of mental and physical suffering. His whole object was to find an antidote, a specific for

29

each and every ailment which could and would drive out the intruder, as though the disorder were a creature of intelligence. In his desire to free himself from affliction and prolong his existence, he has searched the heavens above, he has gone into the deep blue sea, the bowels of the earth, and every portion thereof. He has tried animal and mineral poisons, penetrated the dark forest with superstitious rites and incantations, has gathered herbs, barks, and roots for medicinal uses. In his frenzy for relief, trusting that he might find a panacea, or at least a specific, he has slaughtered man, beast, and bird, making use of their various parts alive and dead. He has made powders, ointments, pills, elixirs, decoctions, tinctures, and lotions of all known vegetables and crawling creatures which could be found, giving therefor his reasons according to his knowledge.

"One question was always uppermost in my mind in my search for the cause of disease. I desired to know why one person was ailing and his associate, eating at the same table, working in the same shop, was not. Why? What difference was there in the two persons that caused one to have pneumonia, catarrh, typhoid or rheumatism, while his partner, similarly situated, escaped. Why?" That is a question that has intrigued many throughout the ages.

D. D. Palmer had plenty of companions in his search for the answer and has plenty to this day. Palmer's personal search was conducted in many fields; for example, he investigated carefully the infant science of osteopathy, founded in 1874, which held that the cause of disease was in the circulation of the blood. Restore normal circulation of blood, said the osteopaths, and the body will cure itself. Although recognizing the importance of blood circulation, Palmer felt that this approach did not deal with the basic inherent forces of the body.

As was pointed out, the healing arts during the latter part of the nineteenth century were in a constant state of flux and confusion. So-called "magnetic healing" came into vogue, dealing with the "unseen forces" of the body. These were defined, not as magical or miraculous, but rather as subtle, invisible energies capable of being felt by others. An example cited by the proponents of this theory was the feeling of ease or lack of ease in the presence of certain people.

Utilizing these principles, with certain manual contacts on different parts of the body, Palmer practiced this art at Burlington, Iowa, and later at Davenport, Iowa.

His success was amazing, a fact which must have pleased him, for healing had its financial ups and downs in those days—at one time he had been forced to make his living by running a grocery store at What Cheer, Iowa.

There were good reasons for Palmer's success with ills of mental origin. Palmer achieved a multitude of cures and patients flocked to him in droves.

Palmer's appearance, too, was striking. He was a short, solidly built man, with jet-black hair and piercing black eyes, who literally exuded energy. His full ebon beard gave him a patriarchal impressiveness, and he was also somewhat of a dandy, wearing a broad-brimmed sombrero and driving a spanking pair of thoroughbred horses. To top it off, he was a remarkable personality.

Palmer maintained an elaborate office in a Davenport building which employed a Negro janitor named Harvey Lillard, who was quite deaf. He could not hear the noise of rigs in the street below and people had to shout at him in order to make themselves heard.

On September 18, 1895, Lillard was tidying up in Palmer's office.

"How long have you been deaf, Harvey?" D. D. shouted.

"Over seventeen years," replied Lillard.

This, to Palmer, was worth investigating, for people who have heard at some time in their lives do not go deaf without cause. "How did it happen?" he asked. "What brought it on, Harvey? Do you know?"

Lillard explained that one day, while he was at work, he had bent down in a stooped position. Suddenly he felt and also heard something in his back go "pop" and he went deaf almost instantly. He had not been able to hear since.

"Did it hurt at the time?" asked Palmer. "Does it still hurt?"

The answer to both questions was "yes."

"Let me look at your back," Palmer then asked. Lillard took off his shirt. Palmer examined his backbone and discovered a good sized protuberance that was obviously a *misaligned vertebra.*

Gently, Palmer felt the bump, asking as he did so, "Does that hurt, Harvey? Is that where you felt sore right after you heard the popping sound?"

Again the replies were in the affirmative.

"All right, Harvey," Palmer finally said. "Do you mind if I attempt to treat this thing?"

Lillard said he didn't mind.

D. D. told Lillard to lie face downward on the floor, and he complied. Then Palmer gave him a sharp thrust on the protruding bump using the spinal bony extensions as levers. Lillard got up and almost immediately he said that he could hear a little better than before.

Nevertheless, his hearing was still far from normal, while the bump remained pronounced. Over the next couple of days, Palmer continued to give a "hand treatment"—Palmer's first term for what he was doing —and reduced the protuberance somewhat, while the man's hearing continued to improve in striking parallel. Within less than a week, the lump was no longer noticeable and Lillard could hear as well as anybody else. Until the time of his death, he had no recurrence of his former deafness.

This was a simple and dramatic example of associating an effect with its cause and then, by eliminating the cause, doing away with the effect, or symptom. It was based on knowledge, inquiry, and experimentation. "There was nothing accidental about this," Palmer wrote himself, "as it was accomplished with an object in view, and the result expected was obtained." He recognized that he had discovered an important way to affect the inherent forces of the body through the nervous system.

It was not long before Palmer discovered he was getting much better results with his "hand treatments," as he continued to dub his manipulation of spinal irregularities, than he had ever realized from his experiments with magnetic healing. He was successful in relieving a wide variety of ailments which had not responded previously to attempts to restore blood circulation or to magnetic healing. His practice grew phenomenally.

The origin of the word "chiropractic" is interesting. One of Palmer's first and highly pleased "hand-treatment" patients was a minister, Rev. Samuel Weed, who was quite a student of Greek. Rev. Weed thought that a distinctive name should be created for what appeared to be a revolutionary and phenomenally successful method of healing, and he told Palmer so.

"What name would you suggest?" asked D. D.

"Why not simply combine the Greek words for 'hand' and 'done by?'" suggested Rev. Weed. Palmer thought it was a good idea, and the word chiropractic —combining *chiro* and *praktikos*—came into existence.

In its early stages, however, chiropractic was as remote from the precise science it is today as Edison's pioneer fiber-filament electric light bulbs were from the modern high-vacuum protected tungsten filaments. But the basic theory has always remained the same. On this foundation the science has grown steadily.

What is this basic chiropractic foundation?

Here we have a few of the fundamental principles of chiropractic as stated by its discoverer, David Daniel Palmer, in his book, *The Science, Philosophy, and Art of Chiropractic:*

"Chiropractic is founded upon the relationship of bones, nerves, and muscles.

"Chiropractic is founded upon the principle that functions receive their vital force through the nervous system. From this fundamental principle, other principles are formed which assist in creating the science and art of chiropractic.

"Displacement of any part of the skeletal frame may press against nerves, which are the channels of communication, intensifying or decreasing their carrying capacity, creating either too much or not enough functionating, an aberration known as disease. The nature of the affection depends upon the shape of the bone, the amount of pressure, age of patient, character of nerves impinged upon, and the individual make-up.

"Chiropractors adjust, by hand, all displacements of the 200 bones, more especially those of the vertebral column, for the purpose of removing nerve impingements which are the cause of deranged functions. The long bones and the vertebral processes are used as levers by which to adjust displacements of osseous tissue of the body. By so doing, normal transmission of nerve-force is restored.

"I think that there is some good in all methods; but when the chiropractor adjusts the bony framework to its normal position, all pliable tissue will respond and resume its proper position and consequently its usual functions—health being the result.

"I have never felt it beneath my dignity to do anything to relieve human suffering."

On the bedrock of Palmer's fundamentals, chiropractic has progressed through the years. It has proven beyond doubt that interference with normal transmission of nerve impulses reduces the living organism's inherent power to heal itself. Most of this interference occurs where the major nerve trunks emerge from the spinal cord through apertures, known as foramina, between the vertebrae of the spinal column. By manual manipulation, the doctor of chiropractic corrects the spinal structural derangement, known as "subluxation." This, in turn, restores normal nerve integration and functioning, and the body's inherent healing powers are enabled to restore health.

If this appears at first thought to be a startling theory, bear in mind that it is no more fantastic than the idea of germs as the cause of disease appeared to many medical men at the time it was first publicized by Pasteur. This is also true of many other developments which at first were widely ridiculed, but later gained universal acceptance. The incredibly complex nervous system, its association with the spine, and the mechanics of spinal subluxations and their correction is the subject of Chapter Five. It will suffice at this point, however, to note that in recent years, the medical profession itself has provided documentation of the theories first advanced by D. D. Palmer.

The famous Dr. Alexis Carrel wrote in his popular book, *Man, the Unknown,* of a mysterious something he called "Natural Health," which he declared "comes from resistance to infectious and degenerative diseases, from equilibrium of the nervous system . . ."

The late Dr. George Crile, one of the greatest of modern medical scientists, wrote that an electrical conductivity flows between the brain and the body, and that when there is a normal flow a "living process" goes on; when there is no flow a "dead process" is in effect. The intermediate condition is a "partial flow" which causes a "disease process." Dr. Crile declared that through laboratory experiments he had been able to locate interferences in the spine that cause "partial flow."

Along the same lines, Dr. David Riesman, Professor of the History of Medicine at the University of Pennsylvania, wrote recently, "Not only has the newer nerve physiology revealed electrical activities and chemical changes in nerves carrying impulses that were scarcely suspected a few years ago, but lately, by ingenious apparatus, electrical forces have been revealed in the brain. It would appear as if all vital processes were in the last analysis electrical."

In the pages of the *American Journal of Medical Science,* Dr. H. T. Hyman gave as one of the reasons for the popularity of chiropractors "the failure of the medical profession to provide this type of service." In *Therapeutic Review,* Dr. M. C. King wrote, "The sooner the medical profession recognizes the work of the chiropractor, the better."

In the *New York State Medical Journal,* Dr. G. W. Hensen described the case of a patient who had been told at a medical hospital that he had a crushed vertebra. This patient went to a chiropractor. He was suffering severe pain in his back and in the back of his left leg and thigh. "It improved under treatment," Dr. Hensen wrote, "and by June 15 (the patient had started chiropractic in April), the pain in the thigh and leg had disappeared and the pain in the back was less intense."

Not long ago the noted medical writer Dr. William Brady devoted a full newspaper column to a description of the way in which a chiropractor "friend" had quickly cured a patient of a knee ailment which had failed to improve after many months of medical treatment. Somewhat reprovingly, Dr. Brady addressed a few words directly to his own medical colleagues: "In short, fellows, here's a darn chiropractor who deserves recognition as a healer, a physician, and if we regulars would rid our minds of a few of the quaint prejudices that linger and invite all healers to join in one big healers' guild or association, it would be a great step for medicine, healing, or whatever you please to call the doctor business."

Overseas, in *British Medical and Surgery Journal,* Osgood and Morrison have referred frankly to "brilliant and rapid . . . chiropractic cures."

One of the most dramatic instances of very great medical interest in chiropractic occurred in Germany in 1953. Five thousand medical doctors were attending the German Therapy Week Convention at Karlsruhe, in Western Germany. One of the principal speakers was a medical doctor, Dr. Karl Sell, Chief of Staff at the famous Orthopedic Sanatarium for Athletes at Allgau, and also an investigator of nonmedical methods of healing. Dr. Sell had made a thorough study of chiropractic, and he was enthusiastic about it. Among other things, he told the assembled M.D.'s that chiropractors possess specialized training which makes them experts on the anatomy of the body, the spinal column in particular. He reminded them of the devastating remark of the famous Swiss professor and doctor, Prof. Bircher-Brenner, who said bluntly, "Up to now I have not yet met one M.D. who could judge the spinal column half as well as a competent chiropractor." Dr. Sell stated that chiropractic can and does cure by restoring the spinal vertebrae to their proper positions.

"The value of chiropractic," Dr. Sell stressed, "is to be found not only in its curative powers, but also in its ability to keep health up to par. Every person, even when in seemingly good health, can benefit from regular chiropractic adjustments (repositionings of displaced vertebrae) since they will improve circulation, remove interference with the nervous system, and help him to enjoy life to a fuller extent."

At the end of his talk, Dr. Sell recommended to the 5,000 physicians that their patients receive regular chiropractic care. The very next morning a long line of medical doctors was waiting at Dr. Sell's door for personal chiropractic attention.

CHAPTER FOUR

A Visit to a Chiropractor

If you are visiting a chiropractor for the first time, the chances are that you are already ill and that medical science has failed to help you. And you have probably heard about chiropractic in one of the following ways.

You have been recommended to a chiropractor by a satisfied chiropractic patient. In this case, chiropractic has probably been praised to you with such fervor that you may consider it a miraculous cure-all; it is far from that, as chiropractors themselves point out. No responsible method of healing claims to be able to cure everything. Chiropractic has, however, demonstrated amazing success in the treatment of a multitude of ailments which medical science has failed to benefit.

You have perhaps heard of at least one chiropractic cure in considerable detail. If it is a case similar to yours, you approach chiropractic with hope and not as a last desperate expedient. Maybe you know something about chiropractic procedure—you know that the chiropractor does not, as many persons erroneously believe, massage you, wallop your backbone with a mallet or his fist, twist your limbs about, or damage you in any way. You are convinced that chiropractic, even if it fails to benefit your particular condition, can at least do you no harm. Finally, you are equipped with the name of a chiropractor who has been described to you as a competent practitioner. Chiropractors vary in skill just as do medical doctors.

You have been recommended to a chiropractor by a medical doctor. Until recently, this did not happen too often, but now it is happening with increasing frequency. Consider, for example, what happened in the case of Col. George E. Ijams, Director of National Rehabilitation of the Veterans of Foreign Wars, and for twenty-seven years top Assistant Administrator of the Veterans Administration.

Col. Ijams had a medical background; his father, a great uncle, and three cousins were M.D.'s. He had a neck condition that medical doctors had diagnosed as neuritis. A man who was not only a medical doctor but a medical administrator as well said to him, "George, would you like to get rid of that discomfort you are suffering from?"

When Col. Ijams answered that he certainly didn't want to keep it, the medical administrator said frankly, "For heaven's sake don't tell anyone I ever suggested this to you, but if you want to get rid of it, go down to the man I go to because I have the identical complaint and he is the only man in this town who has given me any relief." He gave the colonel the name of a chiropractor.

The reaction of Col. Ijams was similar to that of many to whom chiropractic is recommended for the first time. As he put it, "Having been raised in a medical atmosphere, I thought that it was a sort of sacrilege to talk about a chiropractor. So I went down there with a good deal of fear in my heart. But when I walked out of that office, I could turn my head very much better than I could when I came in. After the second treatment, I had no more neuritis."

Your medical doctor has condemned chiropractic to you. This happens very frequently, as Dr. Horace Gray noted somewhat caustically in *New International Clinics*: "It is well known that the regular physician seldom speaks favorably in public of any doctor outside the regular fold." Bear in mind that it is the exceptional medical doctor who knows anything about chiropractic. It is not taught in medical schools, it is seldom mentioned favorably in medical journals, and it is frequently belittled in these same areas. The average medical doctor, in giving what he believes to be an honest appraisal of chiropractic, may call it "unscientific," "crackpotish," or even "sheer quackery." He may admit that, "It's good in a few cases of back-ache, but that's about all."

When an M.D. expresses such an opinion, one might ask him, "Then how do you explain the fact that there are more than thirty-five million chiropractic patients today in this country alone and that their number is increasing at a rate of two million a year?" In attempting to answer this he will probably reveal his own ignorance of chiropractic.

You have read items about chiropractic in the public press or the popular magazines. These may be articles extolling chiropractic or perhaps condemning it. Nevertheless, you have obtained sufficient information to stimulate you to investigate further.

A Visit to a Chiropractor

You have merely heard about chiropractic in a vague way, know nothing about it, but are trying it as a "last desperate resort."

However you may have heard about chiropractic, once you have decided that you are "going to try a chiropractor," the first and most important thing you will want to know is, "How can I be sure that I will select a good one?"

If a chiropractor has already been highly recommended to you, there's no problem. If not, you can make inquiries just as you would about the merits of medical doctors. Few towns are so small that they do not have at least one chiropractor. Find out who a few of the local chiropractic patients are and ask questions of them. In towns of any considerable size, good sources of information are union leaders, shop foremen, and other employed persons who deal with groups of people of considerable size.

As in the case of medical doctors, there are chiropractic associations and groups whose members must meet rigid professional standards in order to belong. In all states where the practice of chiropractic is regulated by law, chiropractors must pass state administered examinations before being permitted to practice their profession. Find out about the chiropractic organization in your area and query it.

Like medical doctors, the doctor of chiropractic is thoroughly trained in all methods of diagnosis. In the physical examination of the patient, he makes a skillful analysis of the spinal column for body balance, postural distortions, and spinal defects which may be causing nerve irritation and resultant dysfunction. A careful examination of all skeletal structures and the nervous system is indeed an important factor in his diagnosis.

In addition, he may use in his diagnosis all modern laboratory and clinical procedures, such as electrocardiography, stethoscopy, percussion, auscultation, nerve tracing, urinalysis, blood tests, blood-pressure instruments, X-ray diagnosis, and other scientific instruments and procedures, as indicated.

In fact, the diagnostic value of the X ray has played a very vital part in chiropractic's continuing research into the causes of diseases which stem from spinal defects, postural distortions, occupational hazards, and the stresses and strains of "high pressure" living, which produce constant tension and nerve irritation. These irritations can upset the functioning of the various bodily organs, conditions which may result in far more serious disease, if not promptly corrected.

Your chiropractor will depend very greatly on his highly trained and sensitive fingers in performing his analysis. He will examine your spine digitally with great care, noting the various curves and irregularities that are detectable by touch; this is known as palpation. In addition, when he locates an area that is sensitive, that reveals tenderness, pain, or that may even be numb, he will determine its extent and then follow the course of the nerve or nerves leading to or from it by means of his fingers; this is termed "nerve tracing."

Nerve tracing can also be done by means other than the fingers alone; there are various extremely sensitive devices which some chiropractors use to aid them in this part of the analysis. One of these is the neurocalometer—the name means simply "nerve heat meter." It takes full advantage of the fact that nerves whose transmission of impulses are hampered in some way throw off an abnormal amount of heat.

An advanced method for detecting spinal hyperemia, caused by nerve irritation, is done electronically by means of a photoelectric device.

Another means of locating nerve interference is by picking up minute electric currents from the tissues. A variety of instruments is used for this purpose.

These are only a few of the devices employed in chiropractic for detecting structural and nervous abnormalities within the body. For many conditions these instruments are not required, and if you are an average patient, you may never get to know much about any of them.

In addition to palpation with the fingers, which is extremely revealing, your chiropractor may have you stand in front of an ordinary plumb line and ask you to turn this way and that while he looks for evidences of curvatures of spine and shoulders, tilting of the head to one side, and other irregularities.

By the time your chiropractor has completed his physical examination and arrived at his analysis of where the nerve impingement or other interference is and what vertebrae are causing it and in just what way, you should have a pretty good idea of why Prof. Bircher-Brenner said, "Up to now I have not yet met one M.D. who could judge the spinal column half as well as a competent chiropractor."

Once he has determined the area that requires attention, the chiropractor will initiate you into the "adjustment." In this process he is seeking to correct an interference with nerve impulses. He does this by moving a vertebra in the direction necessary to realign it to normal position, and restore normal nerve function.

To perform his work, the chiropractor will have to overcome the tension of the body, increased probably by the uncertainty and even fear which you may feel.

The fairly immediate reactions to your "adjustment" may be none or several. You may feel exhilarated, you may experience a sensation of warmth throughout your body or in one specific area. After all, nerve function has been altered for the better. It takes the nerve control center a little while to become accustomed to the new situation and restore normal function.

Although the doctor of chiropractic is primarily concerned with the relationship between structural anatomy and health, his four years of training at chiropractic college prepare him to deal with the patient as a distinct personality as well as a physical organism. Thus mental and emotional problems, as well as physical complaints, form the basis for treating the whole person. He places reliance on the inherent recuperative powers of the human body and patient managment is conducted with due regard to environmental, nutritional, and psychotherapeutic factors, as well as to first aid, hygiene, sanitation, rehabilitation, and related procedures designed to restore and maintain normal nerve function.

CHAPTER FIVE

Man's Incredible Nervous System

"The human brain is the most powerful embodiment of electromagnetic energy of which we have any knowledge."

This fundamental fact was so expressed by the Englishman, Francis Grierson, and appeared in the *Westminster Review*. Its immense truth is becoming more and more apparent every day as increasingly delicate and precise means of studying the structure and the workings of the brain come into existence.

Within the brain's 1,350 or so cubic centimeters of gray and white matter lie inestimable billions of neurons or nerve cells. It has been hazarded roughly that there are more than *fourteen billion* such cells in the cerebral cortex or outer layers of the upper, conscious brain alone. If all its possible neuron connections were utilized in a manner identical with the laying out of all possible combinations of playing cards, for example, the brain would achieve more "thought combinations," no two of them identical, than there are stars in the entire universe!

It has been said that man can never hope to build an electronic brain capable of duplicating the capacities of the human brain for the simple reason that such a machine would require the power of many Niagaras while the space required to house it would be many cubic miles. Thus the idea that "robot brains" will ever replace thinking man is absurd.

D. D. Palmer was ridiculed widely when he first expressed the thought that the normally functioning brain, operating through a sound nervous system, regulates and integrates every body activity down to the workings of the tiniest cell. He called this capacity "innate intelligence."

Palmer was far ahead of his time. Today his theory has been amply proven and is almost universally accepted. One of the most vivid descriptions of the immense executive powers of the brain was written by the late Dr. Frank Crane and it is both highly picturesque and accurate:

"The smartest man in the world is the Man Inside. By the Man Inside I mean that Other Man within each of us that does most of the things we give ourselves credit for doing. You may refer to him as Nature or the Subconscious Self, or think of him as merely a Force or a Natural Law or, if you are religiously inclined, you may use the term God . . .

"I say that he is the smartest man in the world. I know he is infinitely more clever and resourceful than I am or any other man is that I ever heard of. When I cut my finger it is he that calls up the little phagocytes to come and kill the septic germs that get into the wound and cause blood poisoning. It is he that coagulates the blood, stops the gash, and weaves the new skin . . . No living man knows enough to make

48

toenails grow, but the Man Inside thinks nothing of growing nails and teeth and thousands of hairs all over my body; long hairs on my head and little fuzzy ones over the rest of the surface of the skin . . . Most of our happiness, as well as our struggles and misery, comes from the Man Inside . . ."

Detailed knowledge of the extent to which the brain is capable of controlling the most minute bodily parts and processes has been achieved only recently. It has come from precise study of the working of the brain not only in health but in sickness as well. With instruments like the electroencephalograph the various brain waves and their rhythms under varying circumstances have been observed as, for example, the "electrical storms" that occur in the brains of epileptics. With devices like the so-called "lie detector" the influence of the emotions upon such functions as pulse, blood pressure, rate of breathing, and production of perspiration has been noted. There has been much study of the effect of brain tumors and other brain injuries. Much work has been done on the brains of animals.

Remove a tiny portion of the hypothalamus or brain stem of a cat and his heartbeat slows, his temperature and blood pressure fall, and he sleeps the remainder of his life. A similar effect can be produced by applying an electric current to the same area.

The anolis lizard is quite a remarkable animal in that he is able to change the color of his skin in accordance with the color of his surroundings. Remove his pituitary gland, however, and he turns a bright green and remains that shade permanently. The protective function that once was able to alter the color of millions of surface cells in unison no longer exists.

Brain tumors can cause a multitude of symptoms ranging from blurred vision to paralysis. Just a few of them are hiccoughs, headaches, failure of speech and memory, epilepsy, abnormal acuteness of the senses, vomiting, the faithful mimicking of a wide variety of diseases including syphilis, heart trouble, nephritis, and indeed disturbances anywhere in the body.

If the posterior lobe of the brain is badly damaged, the awareness of fear with all its attendant defenses such as stepped-up metabolism and production of adrenalin are lost. Injuries to the brain sometimes produce even more bizarre symptoms. A man who was hit on the right side of the head with a block of wood promptly developed an abnormal thirst, drinking as much as thirty-two and one-half pints of water in a single day. The symptom gradually declined as the brain healed and in about two weeks the man was drinking normal quantities of water as before. A soldier was shot above the right ear. Formerly his behavior had been excellent and he had been a teetotaller, but now he became insubordinate and a drunkard besides. An oil feeder spout was accidentally driven into a railroad fireman's brain above his right eye; much of his left side became paralyzed and memory of the previous twenty years was totally wiped out. A man injured on the right side of the head developed auditory hallucinations and epileptic fits and finally murdered an entire family.

Following an automobile accident in which the back of his head was bumped, a man developed sinusitis, numbness of the muscles, and arthritis. A boy received a bump on his head while playing "touch ball" and instantly went deaf. Two weeks later he was bumped on the head again and regained his hearing.

These are just a few of the multitudinous symptoms that can and frequently do follow brain injuries. They demonstrate some of the ill effects that can be produced in various parts of the body and indeed throughout the entire body by a brain that is not functioning normally.

What are the beneficial effects that may be expected from a brain that is functioning properly and that is "getting its signals through" to all parts of the body?

In attempting to answer this question another question might well be posed: "What is the secret of natural immunity?"

That a natural immunity exists in some of us possibly all of the time, and perhaps in all of us at least some of the time, has been demonstrated beyond doubt. But the reason for this remains to the vast majority as much of an enigma today as it was to D. D. Palmer when he "desired to know why one person was ailing and his associate, eating at the same table, working in the same shop, was not . . ."

Here is a portion of that enigma. In the deadliest epidemic of all time, the "Black Plague" of the mid-14th Century, an estimated fifty per cent of the population of the then known world were stricken and of those who contracted the plague almost all died. Yet half of the population were mysteriously not stricken, although the bubonic bacilli could enter the system via the nose or mouth or a mere scratch on the skin. What saved this other half?

Probably every person contains some tubercle bacilli at some time or another during his lifetime. When cadavers are autopsied, almost invariably lesions typical of tuberculosis are found. Yet few of us ever reveal the symptoms of tuberculosis, while only a small minority are seriously attacked by the disease.

The antibodies of poliomyelitis exist in almost everyone, indicating that the germs have been active in most of us, yet few ever show even the slightest symptoms of polio.

Following an epidemic of typhoid in Croydon, England, the British bacteriologist, Hugh Nicol, asked plaintively in his book *Microbes by the Millions,* "The question that is still unsolved is not why did tens die and hundreds fall ill, but why did thousands fail to get the disease?"

And, according to Dr. Lars F. Gulbrandtsen of the University of Illinois there is no such thing as a "germ-free" person. Every human being contains the germs of disease in his blood and tissues within a few minutes after birth.

There is amazing evidence that the properly functioning body contains within itself all the resources it requires to combat successfully the development of any and all disease. It produces its own germicidal agents; the skin itself kills germs better than the majority of antiseptics. The mucous membranes secrete germ killers and the gastric and intestinal juices contain germicides. If inimical germs get into the blood stream specialized blood cells go after them and destroy them or render them harmless in some way or other.

Consider what happens in the healthy body when

tuberculosis germs are present, for example. Macrophages or "wandering" germ-destroying cells are produced in enormous quantities, seek out the bacteria, surround and devour them. Thriving on their choice diet of germs, the macrophages develop far beyond their normal size and build living walls around the bacteria with their bodies, thus depriving the attackers of oxygen and nourishment. If ulceration occurs, scar tissue forms, providing a further barrier. Enzymes and hormones of various sorts also aid in the battle.

The efficiency with which the healthy body attacks and destroys disease germs is dramatically demonstrated in the case of meningitis, which has been carefully studied during epidemics. It is an inflammatory disease of the brain and spinal cord and very often it is lethal. During a meningitis epidemic, examination of any 1,000 persons selected at random will reveal that from 50 to 200 of the group have the potentially deadly meningococci in their bodies. But if these same 1,000 persons are examined the very next day, it is not unlikely that most or many who harbored the germs the day before will be entirely free of meningococci.

Thus D. D. Palmer's "innate intelligence" or Dr. Crane's "Man Inside" is a very efficient fighter of disease provided he is able to marshal his forces and get them to where they are needed. But to do this, the brain must tell him just what is going on and where and just what sort of defense is needed and in what degree. Otherwise there is no such thing as "natural immunity" or "resistance to disease." As Dr. Crile noted, when there is only a "partial flow" of electrical messages between the brain and the body a "disease process" is able to exist.

The human brain is of fantastic complexity for a very simple reason. It is, or is intended to be, the dictator of every cell and function of the body. It is not surprising therefore that its communications system, the nervous system, is also fantastically complex.

Perhaps the most graphic description of the thoroughness with which the nervous system permeates the entire body was written for *Morris' Human Anatomy* by Dr. Irving Hardesty, professor of anatomy at Tulane University. "So intimate and extensive is the distribution (of nerves) throughout the body," stated Dr. Hardesty, "that could all the other tissues be dissolved away, still there would be left in gossamer its form and proportions—a phantom of the body composed entirely of nerves."

The nervous system somewhat resembles an inverted tree, whose trunk stems downward from the base of the brain and whose tiniest twig endings are in the cells. Its "main line" is of course the spinal cord which is silvery colored and about as thick as the little finger. The spinal cord is in essence a secondary brain, a cable of millions of living wires performing the same function as a telephone trunk line with this important difference: there is no two-way transmission on any given wire. Some of the wires handle only "incoming" messages to the brain while others handle only "outgoing" messages to the various areas and units of the body. The nerves leading to the brain are known as "afferent" or inward in direction of their transmission; the nerves leading from the brain are known as "efferent" or outward transmitting.

Like branches emanating from the trunk of a tree, smaller nerve cables lead from the spinal cord at intervals along its length. They emerge through openings or foramina between the vertebrae of the spinal column, and they emerge in pairs, one to the left and one to the right. This mechanism is extremely intricate and will be described later in this chapter.

Every afferent or incoming nerve has its beginning in a highly specialized information-gathering device which is called a "receptor end organ." These receptors are located throughout the body, in the skin, subcutaneous tissues, hair follicles, muscles, tendons, ligaments, cartilages, joints, capsules, periosteum, and all viscera. Each, according to its function, picks up information concerning such important items as temperature, light, pressure and other sensations.

The total number of receptor end organs in the entire body is probably incalculable. In the skin alone there are millions which are sensitive only to heat and cold. Millions more that are light sensitive are clustered in the eyes. In the taste buds are additional millions which are sensitive to sweet, sour, and bitter.

Ultimately every bit of information that is picked up by the receptor end organs goes into a "weather report" that reaches the brain, where it is processed. If action of some sort is necessary, instructions are sent to the appropriate destinations via the efferent or outgoing nerves.

Some idea of the complexity of this process may be gained from the fact that in the performance of even the simplest act or function, such as yanking a hand away from a hot stove or blinking an eye, the incoming and outgoing impulses travel over millions of separate nerve connections, being "switched" to their proper destinations by some master selective device whose nature one cannot even remotely begin to guess.

Almost invariably, the instructions sent out by the brain are far more complicated than are the incoming bits of information and require the employment of far more nerves and nerve connections. This in itself would seem to prove that in the brain is centered the control of everything that goes on in the body. Conclusive anatomical proof exists, too, in the overwhelmingly greater numbers of outgoing nerves as compared with incoming ones. At each spinal foramina, for example, there are somewhere between 100,000 and 150,000 cables that carry outgoing messages from the brain. By contrast there are only about 40,000 cables that carry incoming messages. All are bound together at this point in one super-cable which, however, is still much slimmer than the spinal cord.

Here a very puzzling question is likely to arise: If the brain controls all bodily processes, how is it that the adjustment of a spinal vertebra, as in the case of Harvey Lillard, can effect any improvement in an ailment existing above that vertebra, as Lillard's deafness? For that matter, how can an adjustment at any point in the spine below the region that is ailing correct the condition above?

The answer is found in the structure and functions of a specialized branch of the nervous system known as the *sympathetic system* which is connected with the incoming and outgoing spinal nerves but is also entirely distinct in itself.

The sympathetic system consists of two strings of ganglia or groups of nerve cells, one on each side of the spinal column. Its first ganglion or knot of cells located in the upper part of the spine sends nerve fibers to the nerves of the cranium and indeed to all organs of the head. Impulses from these fibers control the secretion of all glands and the blood supply to the various organs in the head.

However, this topmost ganglion of the sympathetic system, called the *superior cervical,* also connects with all four of the topmost nerves emanating from the spine. Because of this fact, a subluxation of spinal vertebrae can seriously interfere with the functioning of the ganglion and in turn with various functionings of the head, even though the subluxation is below the head. In effect, the ganglion is serving as a shunt. Subluxations much farther down the spine can also affect the head due to the fact that there are superior cervical connections in that area as well.

The brain itself can also be adversely affected by subluxations of the spine. Although both the brain and the spinal cord are sheathed by a continuous membrane, they have different sources of blood supply. Interference with the functioning of any of the spinal nerves which emanate from between the vertebrae and then re-enter the vertebral canal to innervate or energize the blood vessels there, may in turn adversely affect brain functioning. Finally, a subluxation in the upper neck region which causes pressure upon the vertebral arteries leading upward to the brain may also be detrimental to the brain.

These and other complexities in the nervous system explain such peculiar phenomena as "referred pain" in which an injury, malfunctioning, or disease condition is felt not where it actually exists but somewhere else. They also explain how a brain that is not working properly or that is getting its signals incorrectly can produce all manner of false symptoms anywhere in the body. And they explain that eeriest of all sensations—feeling a portion of the body that is no longer a part of it, such as a leg that has been amputated.

To understand just how gravely spinal subluxations can affect the transmission of nerve impulses to and fro along the spinal cord and the great nerve cables emanating therefrom, it is necessary to have some knowledge of the spinal column itself.

This "interlocking chain of bones" known as the spine is a marvelously complicated and efficient structure which performs a multitude of duties so effortlessly that we are seldom aware of them. Yet a moment's thought will make it clear that, among other things, the spine supports and balances the head, supports the arms and serves as a fulcrum for them, partially supports the trunk, serves as a vertical spring which absorbs shocks such as those incurred in walking, serves as a flexible mechanism that coordinates a vast variety of bodily activities such as walking, stooping and twisting, and supports and protects the spinal cord and its emanating nerves.

Just how intricate and successful an engineering accomplishment the spinal column is was beautifully expressed in *Men in Structure and Function* by Dr. Fritz Kahn:

"If an engineer were given a job of constructing the vertebral column—a flexible column consisting of 33 rings with 150 joints and almost 1,000 ligamentary connections capable of supporting a load of 500 pounds, and yet flexible and elastic—he would perhaps solve the problem tolerably well after a number of years of activity. Yet he would not be able to equal or surpass the work of Nature. If on the day when he delivered his work, the further task was suggested to him of installing the spinal cord within the vetebral column, that is, of laying a nerve cord consisting of millions of wires that pass out between the rings and are not injured in the least by any normal movements of the spinal column itself or the body as a whole, the engineer would certainly consider the suggestion the plan of a madman . . ."

The spine is all the more amazing because, like everything else in nature and in fact throughout this constantly changing universe, it is in a state of evolution, of changing from one form into another. In the case of the spine, the change is from the horizontal to the vertical. Millions of years ago our ancestors crawled upon their bellies; today we are standing erect, although not perfectly so. Ultimately our spines will be perfectly adapted to erect posture, but now they have several pronounced curves caused by the stress of assemblies to whose weight the body has not yet fully adapted. There is a cervical curve caused by the weight of the head not being balanced squarely atop the spine but rather hung somewhat forward (the word *cervical*, of course, stems quite simply from *cervix*, which means "neck," while *anterior* means "forward" or toward the front). A little farther downward is the thoracic, posterior curve; it bends backward under the weight of the ribs and the organs suspended within the chest.

Still farther downward comes the lumbar curve, which is anterior due to the forward pull of the lower belly weight (*lumbus* incidentally means loin). Finally comes the pelvic curve in which the spine bends sharply rearward again.

So it is obvious that our spines are by no means ideal vertical supports and that their development is still going on. For example, our spines are shortening while some of the lower vertebrae are in the process of fusing together to provide more rigid support. Our legs are lengthening. The shorter spine of the future will eliminate the bulging abdomen, the hernia, and the prolapsed uterus, as well as many other mechanical ills to which we are presently so prone. Other mechanical improvements now underway will also prove of great benefit. For instance, the fusion of certain bones in the feet will eliminate fallen arches. The fact that these improvements, particularly in the spine, are still far from complete accounts for a great many of the bodily ills to which we are now subject.

Very simply, the spine consists of an assembly of twenty-four vertebrae. These comprise what we popularly refer to as the backbone. Below these twenty-four vertebrae is the sacrum, which is a part of the pelvic "sacroiliac arrangement" in which a multitude of aches and pains originate. The tail bone below is the coccyx.

While the structures of the individual vertebrae vary, basically they consist of solid disks of bone from which bony protrusions or "processes" extend to the sides and rear and give the spine its characteristic bumpy feeling. These processes fulfill the function of a bony cage which encloses and protects the spinal cord. Examination of any two adjoining vertebrae will reveal semicircular openings in the processes of both that extend to right and left. It is these openings which allow for the passage of the nerves outward from the spinal cord even though the processes themselves are pressed tightly together.

Chiropractors hold that if the vertebrae of the spine are in proper alignment, then the semicircular openings in any two adjoining vertebrae will coincide to provide full circular openings even as the spine is bent and twisted in the normal activities of living, and there will be no interference with the emerging nerves. They also emphasize that if the spinal vertebrae are not properly aligned, the nerves issuing through the foramina will be compressed, stretched, twisted or otherwise distorted.

In particular, they stress that such derangements are almost inevitable in our highly unnatural way of living which necessitates prolonged repetition of mechanical activities or compels many of us to sit in the same constrained position for hours on end. These derangements begin in childhood when many of us develop a "postural slouch" that persists throughout life. For adults there is a whole battery of occupational requirements that tend to throw the spine out of line and make the body sick. Some ailments resulting from various occupations even have descriptive names, such as "typist's neck" and "policeman's feet" (flat-feet). There is a "railroad back" and even a "jazz spine" which afflicts hot drummers. The new dance craze, "The Twist," may damage the spine. There is a "housewife's backache" and a "pianist's slouch." There are "one-handed occupations" that produce their own distinctive symptoms. In particular, participants in a wide variety of sports such as baseball, bowling, golf, and tennis often pay for their fun with specialized aches and pains. Butchers, carpenters, engineers, farmers, mailmen, mechanics, painters, plasterers, plumbers, printers, and tailors all have their own peculiar ills.

It is quite obvious that in the normal course of everyday activities the vertebrae of the spine would grind and even bump against each other constantly unless Nature had taken some precaution to cushion these shocks. Imagine, for instance, the wear and tear on the solid disks, processes, spinal cord, and emerging nerves that would occur in even so simple and common a pastime as playing ball with a child or hopping about in a game of leap-frog. The noise would probably resemble the proverbial skeletons dancing on a tin roof. Fortunately, cushions have been provided in the form of disks of tough yet elastic cartilage—known as the intervertebral disks—which separate the solid, supporting disks of the spine. There is also cushioning where the nerves emerge from the spinal cord between the processes. This cushioning, however, is unable to protect either the bones or the nerves properly when the spinal bones themselves are out of line.

There are, incidentally, many other cushions located at points of friction, shock, pressure, torque, and so on throughout the body. The best known of these are the bursae. Anybody who has experienced the pain of bursitis knows what happens when they are not functioning properly.

To repeat, chiropractic holds that by the correction of structural misalignments in the body, for the most part in the spinal column, interferences with the nervous system are eliminated and the body is enabled to cure itself. It may come as a surprise to many to learn that spinal adjustment as a very effective health restorer in many areas of illness is by no means new, although it is only beginning to be "discovered" by the medical profession today.

CHAPTER SIX

Spinal Manipulation Through the Ages

The person who first observed that "there is nothing new under the sun" has probably been with his ancestors for a long, long time. In all fields of human activity we probably progress more through new combinations and reshufflings of knowledge than by so-called flashes of genius. So it was with chiropractic.

To give D. D. Palmer his full due, healing by various forms of manipulation is actually very ancient and close to universal. It was originally known as the "laying on of hands," and it was practiced not only by the ancient Greeks but also by the Egyptians, Babylonians, Assyrians, Chinese, Tibetans, and Hindus, as well as by the ancient Aztecs and Incas of Central and South America. Such manipulation, however, was a far cry from the specific, localized spinal adjustment developed by Palmer. Moreover, Palmer's realization that nerve interference, and not some other mysterious derangement, lay at the root of disease was entirely new.

Palmer himself admitted frankly that the spinal manipulation which he developed and expanded had originated with the ancients. He emphasized repeatedly that he was not the first person to replace displaced vertebrae, and that the art had been practiced "for thousands of years." However, he did insist that he was the first, both in ancient or modern times, to adjust displaced vertebrae by using the protruding processes as levers for the purpose of *removing pressure from nerves*. And he asserted that from this "basic fact" he had created a new science "destined to revolutionize the theory and practice of the healing art." To this day localized spinal adjustment to remove nerve disturbance has remained the basis of chiropractic although there have been vast improvements in both techniques and the body of knowledge available.

The closest ancient approach to modern chiropractic was probably developed by the ancient Greeks. Hippocrates, the Father of Healing and the greatest clinician of all time, stated flatly that "physical structure is the basis of medicine" and went into great detail concerning the importance to health of a well-adjusted spine.

"One or more vertebrae of the spine may or may not go out of place very much," Hipprocrates warned. "They might give way very little, and, if they do, they are likely to produce serious complications and even death, if not properly adjusted . . . It appears to me that one ought to know what diseases arise in man from the powers, and what from the structures. By powers I mean intense and strong juices, and by the structures, whatever conformations there are in men . . . The spinal marrow would suffer if from the displacement of a vertebra it were to be bent even to a small extent, for the displaced vertebra would compress the spinal marrow if it did not break it; and, if compressed and strangled, it would induce insensibility of many great and important parts. Many diseases are related to the spine."

The average layman is amazed at even a partial listing of the ailments in which pronounced benefit and cure have been achieved through chiropractic. It is difficult for him to grasp the paramount importance of the spinal cord and spinal nerves in the control of disease, although he can understand readily enough what happens when an electrical circuit is shorted or grounded. Hippocrates, although he did not know the "electrical" nature of the nervous system, was well aware of the multitude of diverse illnesses that result from spinal distortions, and he prepared a very long list of them which strikingly parallels modern findings. On this Hippocratic list were:

Abnormal bodily development, especially in youth; difficulty in breathing (dyspnoea), pharyngitis, laryngitis; tuberculosis of the lungs and bones (Pott's disease); nephritis and inflammation of the kidneys and bladder, also purulent abscesses; incapacity of sexual functional activity; in advanced age, crises in diseases that are present; quinsy, catarrh, and head colds; bladder inflammation and retention of urine; involuntary urination and evacuation of the bowels; poor circulation of the lower extremities, numbness in the lower limbs, overall debility and torpor; emaciation and hypertrophy.

The Greeks used a multitude of devices for stretching the spine. Some of these resembled medieval instruments of torture. One, for instance, was a tall, upright affair in which the upper part of the patient's body was hauled upward by means of a windlass while the legs were securely restrained by means of a cable secured around the thighs and fastened to the base of the machine. Another consisted of a ladderlike frame suspended vertically from a pulley; the patient was tied to the rungs of this affair and shaken violently up and down. A common practice was to hold newborn babies by the heels and shake them up and down.

Not all the early Greek spinal therapy devices and procedures were as crude as these. Hippocrates, for example, wrote of the use of spinal manipulation tables upon which the patient lay face downward. And he described a method of manual manipulation of the spine: "The operator must be well versed and capable. The physician or anyone else who is strong and not ignorant should place the thenar (palm) of the one hand upon the protuberance and the thenar of the other hand upon the former, to force the vertebra, by a quick jerk, to slip back into its former place."

Centuries after Hippocrates, Galen re-emphasized the importance of spinal manipulation, and gave this astounding advice, ". . . leaving the affected parts alone, you will reach the spine from which you will treat the disease." Yet his findings, too, were largely ignored by orthodox medical science.

Nevertheless, spinal manipulation of various crude sorts was very widespread throughout the centuries preceding Palmer. An important ritual of Oriental ancestor worship was for children to tread back and forth on the weary spines of their parents. Treading upon the spine has also been a long established therapeutic measure among the Maoris of New Zealand, the

Amerindians, and various African tribes. In Mexico the native Indians even today stretch the spines of the sick by a method called *abrazo del ranchero* (the rancher's embrace). Until fairly recently the Hawaiians practiced a form of vertebral adjustment known as *lomi-lomi.*

All these, however, are but hit-or-miss beginnings and experimentations compared with the highly specialized, highly scientific chiropractic that was discovered by D. D. Palmer and has since been consistently improved both by himself and others. The story of the developments in chiropractic has many dramatic moments and is worthy of a chapter in itself.

CHAPTER SEVEN

The Growth of Chiropractic

Over the decades since D. D. Palmer gave Harvey Lillard the series of adjustments which cured Lillard's deafness, chiropractic has flourished like the green bay tree. Some of this growth was almost frightening in its vigor and sometimes too rapid to be orderly. It took quite a while for chiropractic to really grow up, develop a sound body of knowledge and skill, establish rigorous professional standards and a code of ethics for its practitioners, and gain the public confidence and respect it now enjoys.

These growing pains are nothing unusual; in fact, they have occurred in the maturing of all the arts and sciences, including medicine. Before reviewing chiropractic's earlier trials and tribulations, it might be enlightening to make a few comparisons with medicine. Only the bigoted medical doctor with an over exalted opinion of his own infallibility could take offense at them.

One of the most famous of our early medical doctors was a man named Benjamin Rush. A person of many talents, the good Dr. Rush was a member of the original Constitutional Assembly at the time the Declaration of Independence was being considered. A great believer in human rights—in particular the right of free choice—he warned against a possible medical monopoly of healing in these words, "To restrict the art of healing to one class of men and deny equal privileges to others will constitute the Bastille of medical science. All such laws are un-American and despotic."

Dr. Rush believed in heroic methods of treatment. His favorite concoction, which he employed in a multitude of ills, was so powerful that it was known as "Rush's Thunderbolt." Composed of ten grains of jalop and ten of calomel it was taken in one dose, and if the patient survived its impact, his recovery was assured. Medical atom bombs like this were common in those lusty days.

Medicine was a disorganized free-for-all, or very nearly so, at about the time D. D. Palmer discovered chiropractic, and it continued in that state for some time afterward. Since the average medical doctor is very likely to belittle D. D. Palmer as "an ignorant fish peddler" and chiropractic as unscientific, let's look at a few facts about the status of the medical profession not so long ago.

In Palmer's day a peddler and horse trader named John D. Rockefeller could and did double as a traveling "medicine man" without fear of arrest or punishment. Men who called themselves doctors of medicine peddled "sure cures" for everything from piles to women's diseases. Medical doctors—including an early head of the American Medical Association—saw nothing unethical in advertising their skills in the newspapers.

Medical doctors of today stress the high standards

of their education, yet as recently as 1908, the medical education situation in this country was so scandalous that the Carnegie Foundation retained Dr. Abraham Flexner, an educator and not a medical man, to make a special study of the profession. In due time Dr. Flexner reported that "of the 155 medical schools in existence, the schools were essentially private ventures, money-making in spirit and object . . . Income was simply divided among the lecturers who reaped a rich harvest . . . No applicant for instruction who could pay his fee or sign his note was turned down . . . The man who settled his tuition bill was practically assured of a degree, whether he had regularly attended lectures or not." It was not until considerably after World War I that reforms in medical education recommended by Flexner were generally put into effect. Many a highly respected and competent medical doctor in practice today received only a sketchy formal education; he is a good doctor only because he continued studying after his graduation from the so-called medical school, and not because of the training he received there.

Many of the same conditions prevailed in the early days of chiropractic, and chiropractors themselves are the first to admit this. Despite his founding of chiropractic and the immense contributions he made to the later development of the science, D. D. Palmer himself often acted in accordance with the chaotic standards of the day.

Those were the days when medical men frequently kept their pet discoveries "secret" and capitalized on them for all they were worth. Sometimes groups of specialists like the "bone setters" formed exclusive

71

guilds and pooled their knowledge, which they guarded jealously, not even allowing their patients to observe what they were doing.

Fully aware of the revolutionary nature of his new method of healing, D. D. Palmer tried at first to do about the same thing. He sought to keep chiropractic a family secret, or to share it, at best, with only a chosen few who would be willing to pay him well for his knowledge.

Practically everything that ultimately became part of chiropractic had to be learned from scratch. For example, Palmer's amazing deduction of the connection between the nervous system and general health was scarcely suspected at the time, and medical men refused to admit that spinal subluxations even existed. To this day, some die-hards of organized medicine still refuse to do so. Nevertheless, knowledge accumulated so rapidly that D. D. Palmer soon realized that chiropractic could not be kept secret for long, and that if it were to achieve the dignity of a science, it must be taught thoroughly and by reputable institutions. Only two years after his discovery, in 1897, he founded the first chiropractic school, The Palmer School of Chiropractic, in Davenport. Today it is the largest chiropractic institution in the world. But records show that The Palmer School had only one pupil in 1898, three in 1899, two in 1900, and four in 1902. In 1903, enrollment had jumped to more than a dozen, although the chiropractic course lasted for six months.

Early adjustment tables were crude devices. The addition of a nose aperture and padding, the dividing of the table into several sections that could be raised or lowered independently of each other were the beginning of many improvements. It took years, too, to improve the thrust so that it could be delivered with absolute accuracy and delicacy, with full assurance that there would be no injury to the patient and little, if any, pain. Enthusiastic adoption by chiropractors of the X-ray and other delicate methods for accurately locating and defining subluxations, plus a growing body of knowledge about the spine and nervous system, gradually eliminated the earlier crude methods and evolved chiropractic into the complex and precise science it is today.

In every art and science there are a few giants, a sizable group who may contribute little that is original but who are sincere, hard workers, and finally a fringe of "crackpots." Chiropractic has been no exception. D. D. Palmer was a giant, but he was impractical. His son Bartlett Joshua Palmer, born in What Cheer, Iowa, in 1881, and fourteen-years-old when chiropractic was discovered, was also a giant, but a very practical one indeed. Chiropractors generally hold that while D. D. was the "Discoverer of Chiropractic," his son B. J. deserves recognition as the "Developer of Chiropractic."

Like his father, B. J. was largely self-educated. He developed an early interest in the science started by his father. He was one of the four students in The Palmer School of Chiropractic's Class of 1902 and he was one of its earliest graduates.

In 1906, the professional school founded by his father passed into the son's hands, and he, with his bride, Doctor Mabel Heath Palmer, purchased property and began to expand the facilities of the school.

Under B. J., The Palmer School grew and prospered

phenomenally. By 1915—two years after the death of Palmer, Sr.—enrollment had exceeded 800. World War I reduced enrollments somewhat, but in 1918, the first year of peace, the school had 1,882 students. As early as 1910, the school had acquired an X-ray machine. Like the other reputable schools that had already replaced the fly-by-night variety, its curriculum required twelve months of full-time attendance. Among the subjects taught even then were anatomy, physiology, symptomatology, pathology and diagnosis, toxicology, obstetrics, dissection, and the science and philosophy of chiropractic. These are named in detail because of the attempts frequently made by certain medical doctors to disparage chiropractors as poorly educated.

Almost all the pioneer chiropractors were, in a sense, fanatics. Many became chiropractors for the simple reason that they had benefited from chiropractic first hand—often after medicine failed—and they wanted to give others the benefit they themselves had received. They didn't give a hoot whether chiropractic was scorned by the medical fraternity or not, whether it was approved or even heard of by the general public or not. They came from all walks of life, for sickness is no respector of position. Generally, however, they were not "professional persons" when they went into chiropractic; for, human nature being what it is, such well-established individuals are usually inclined to give thought to their own comfortable careers and act accordingly. They are content with becoming boosters rather than active doers. Even in religion, the prominent convert seldom becomes a missionary.

However, as chiropractic gained in respectability

and numbers of patients, while its educational requirements increased in stringency, this situation rapidly improved. By 1920, when chiropractic was only twenty-five years old, the roster of The Palmer School, then numbering 2,000 students, boasted many persons with previous professional backgrounds, including 102 school teachers, 12 ministers, 16 school superintendents, 14 editors and other journalists, 45 musicians, 24 pharmacists, 11 chemists, 7 dentists, 26 Army and Navy officers, 51 nurses, 165 students who had transferred from other schools of various sorts, and an assortment of artists, engineers, physical-training instructors, and stenographers. There were even a few osteopaths, veterinary surgeons, and medical doctors. Thirty foreign nations were represented.

Meanwhile, other chiropractic schools of integrity were rapidly coming into existence. Typical of these was Carver Chiropractic College of Oklahoma City, which was founded in 1906 and which grew to become the second largest institution of its kind in the nation. Carver started with a six-months' course, about all that was necessary at the time, but increased it to nine months two years later. Shortly afterward the school jumped the length of the course to eighteen months, and as early as 1927, was presenting a course of twenty months. Today the school requires four years of resident class instruction totalling more than 4000 hours. This extension of instruction time has been paralleled in all the reputable chiropractic schools.

Meanwhile, other developments in various fields were underway, all of them strong indications that chiropractic was growing up. In many of them B. J. Palmer pioneered personally. He was one of the earliest and most prolific writers on the new science; by 1910 he had authored five books on the subject. In that same year he started a chiropractic magazine which was the parent of the present monthly journal *The Chiropractor*. He was one of the founders and for a time secretary-treasurer of the first chiropractic organization, The Universal Chiropractic Association. He was responsible for the wide-spread adoption of the word "adjustment" in preference to "treatment" to describe what the chiropractor does. And these are only a few of his many innovations and activities.

Dr. B. J. Palmer was probably the most colorful and controversial personality in chiropractic. He traveled extensively to promote the new science, and fought many courageous battles in debate and in court against the determined opposition of organized medicine. He had the gift of delegating responsibility to subordinates he could trust and he utilized this gift superlatively. And he became powerful in many fields other than chiropractic. He headed a number of businesses and enterprises of various sorts, and owned the first radio station west of the Mississippi, licensing it only three months after the first station in the United States received its license in 1922.

At the time of his death, Dr. Palmer was president of the Tri-City Broadcasting Company of Davenport, Iowa, the Central Broadcasting Company of Des Moines, The Palmer School of Chiropractic and the International Chiropractors Association. He was a recipient of the Du Pont Memorial Award for achievement in communications.

On world tours with his wife and son, David, Dr. Palmer purchased many oriental artifacts and many rare curios that are displayed at the school museum at Davenport. He built up the world's largest collection of human bones comprising more than 20,000 specimens and valued at more than $175,000.

Upon the death of B. J. Palmer in May 1961, his son, Dr. David D. Palmer, accepted the challenge and responsibility of helping chiropractic advance to its rightful position among the healing arts.

This third-generation chiropractic leader, born in 1906, has qualified himself by his sincere interest in chiropractic and his splendid educational background at The Palmer School of Chiropractic, University of Pennsylvania, and Harvard University.

The presidents of twelve chiropractic colleges and the heads of the two national chiropractic associations attended the investiture of Dr. David as president of The Palmer College of Chiropractic on August 20, 1961. Several thousand chiropractors from all over the world attended the ceremonies.

Another giant of chiropractic was Willard Carver who made important contributions relative to the mechanical behavior of the spinal column, body mechanics, and posture.

Dr. Willard Carver was born on July 14, 1876, in a small house located about forty rods from Carver Tavern near the junction of Allen's Grove and Maysville Roads, about twelve miles from Davenport, Iowa. When he was two, his family moved to Mahasha County, Iowa, where they resided until the death of Carver's father in 1901. Carver was educated at the Christian College of Oskaloosa, Iowa. He later finished his scientific and literary training at Drake University in Des Moines, Iowa, where he earned his Bachelor of Laws degree.

Willard Carver practiced law for fourteen years thereafter and specialized in negligence work. This led him to study anatomy and physiology which he found to be of assistance in his frequent appearances in court in negligence cases.

In December, 1895, while sitting in his law office in Ochewydan, Iowa, he received a letter from his old friend D. D. Palmer describing his experiment upon Harvey Lillard. During the ensuing years, Carver, still practicing his profession as a lawyer, became very much interested in Palmer's new science and began to formulate his own theories about the science of chiropractic.

Dr. Carver studied chiropractic both with D. D. Palmer and Dr. Charles Ray Parker, who, at that time was running the Parker School at Ottumwa, Iowa. Although there were a number of schools of chiropractic functioning in the early 1900's, Dr. Willard Carver and one L. L. Denny organized a college of chiropractic in Oklahoma City in 1906.

Dr. Carver's contributions to the development of chiropractic are outstanding and widely known—the most important of these were the distortion by compensation studies in which he evaluated the mechanical behavior of the spine and pelvis under all normal and abnormal conditions. From his original studies, which have been substantiated many times over in later years, Carver became convinced that not only spinal subluxations but also distortions of any and all bodily structures create an environment favorable to the development of disease. Certain that man's effort to overcome the constant pull of gravity is in itself responsible for many distortions, he became one of the pioneer advocates of correct posture, which might be called "preventive chiropractic." From his original observations of minute postural and structural faults, largely stemmed the present-day detailed system of chiropractic analysis.

D. D. Palmer, B. J. Palmer, and Willard Carver are often termed the "Trinity of Giants." However, there were other pioneers in chiropractic, men and women who made important contributions to the advancement of the profession.

Here are but a few of these courageous people who have passed away in recent years. Dr. W. A. Budden, President of the Western States College of Chiropractic, who was noted for his splendid work as chairman of the Council on Education of the National Chiropractic Association. He helped raise educational standards and improve chiropractic colleges. Dr. Frank E. Dean, Founder of the Columbia Institute of Chiropractic—a natural-born student and scholar, he conceived of the idea of a chiropractic college which would combine all of the facets of higher education in its curriculum. Dr. Craig M. Kightlinger, Founder and President of the Eastern Chiropractic Institute and President of the Chiropractic Institute of New York— "Kight", as he was affectionately known, was famous for his great enthusiasm for chiropractic and his ability to teach adjusting procedures. Dr. Hugh B. Logan, Founder of the Logan Basic College of Chiropractic— who researched new techniques in straightening distorted spines. He was probably the one most responsible for the widespread use of the 14 x 36 X-ray film, which revealed the full spinal column with a single exposure. He demonstrated that chiropractors could successfully straighten distorted spines. Since 1944, his work had been carried on vigorously by his son, Dr. Vinton F. Logan, whose recent demise is a great loss to the profession. Dr. William C. Schulze, President of the National College of Chiropractic—a medical doctor who discontinued medical practice to devote his full time to chiropractic education and the introduction of a broad view to chiropractic practice. Dr. L. J. Steinbach, President of the Universal Chiropractic College—whose great interest in chiropractic technique led to the development of the vertical X-ray and the origination of the spinal-balance method of examination and adjusting.

Those interested in the history of chiropractic would also recognize the names of countless other people who have played important roles in chiropractic progress.

It is not surprising that these pioneers often quarreled bitterly and could not agree on many points; such quarrels are the rule, and not the exception, in any complex and evolving art or science. Nevertheless, they all agreed on the basic principles of chiropractic—that it is a science and an art of healing which deals with the relationship between structure and function in the human body, particularly the muscular, skeletal, and nervous systems in the restoration and maintenance of health.

As in other professions, there are different ideas as to how this may best be accomplished. Therefore, it is not strange to see chiropractic practice vary from a limited to a broad approach. Although all chiropractors use spinal adjustments as their modus operandi, there is one group of chiropractors who restrict themselves to spinal adjustments only. Some are so specialized that they deal primarily with the two topmost cervical vertebrae, the atlas and the axis, which comprise the assembly supporting the skull. On the other hand, there is a large group of doctors of chiropractic, who not only make corrections in the spinal column, but also, when indicated, in any of the three-hundred articulations of the body. Many doctors of chiropractic use certain drugless adjuncts in addition to specific adjustments. These supplemental aids include the application of heat and cold, electricity, water, diet, exercise and other rehabilitation procedures.

Despite this divergence on details, all chiropractors adhere rigidly to the premise that spinal adjustments are of greatest benefit and base their handling of any case on such manipulative procedures.

It is not surprising, in light of the above, that there is a variety of techniques of spinal adjustment that has evolved gradually over the years. Generally, there are heavy techniques or light techniques which are used, depending upon the patient and the problem presented. But it is the adjustment for the purpose of removing nerve interference to which chiropractic attributes its extraordinary results.

There is also other evidence that chiropractic is now a mature science. One of the most important factors is the present failure to claim that chiropractic cures anything and everything. Some of the early chiropractors made just this claim in their excessive enthusiasm, but as the profession gained in knowledge, experience, and educational requirements, its practitioners have become appropriately precise and accurate in putting forth the benefits of their healing arts.

The educational standards for chiropractic first promulgated by the Palmers and a few other contemporary pioneers, have steadily been increased in scope and quality. Today, there are some eighteen chiropractic colleges in the United States, with a total student capacity in excess of 7,000. The accredited standard of education today is a four-year resident course of 4,040 hours of study. This, by the way, compares favorably with the hours required by the famed Johns Hopkins School of Medicine. Obviously, the approved chiropractic course does not include many subjects taught in medical schools, such as pharmacology, medicine, surgery, and therapeutics. On the other hand, it includes 1,580 hours of purely chiropractic subjects that are not taught in medical schools, in addition to the "basic sciences" that are required of practitioners of both healing arts.

Among the subjects now included in the chiropractic as well as in the medical education are anatomy, chemistry, physiology, pathology and bacteriology, diagnosis and symptomatology. The "minimum course" recommended includes psychology, endocrinology, dermatology, dietetics, pediatrics, gynecology, kinesiology, and obstetrics. In many states, in order to be licensed, chiropractors must pass the same "basic sciences" examination as medical doctors. In addition, they must pass an examination covering their exclusively chiropractic subjects.

The first state law governing chiropractic was passed in Kansas in 1913. Since then, as previously indicated, all but four states of the United States have passed chiropractic practice acts, and it is probable that these four will follow the example of the others in the not too distant future. Also as previously indicated, chiropractic has been recognized by legislative action in numerous foreign countries.

Like medical practice acts, chiropractic practice acts exist for the protection of the public. Among their several objectives are defining the science of chiropractic and describing what services the chiropractor is legally permitted to perform, establishing educational requirements for chiropractors and providing for the examination of candidates for the chiropractic license, granting licenses to chiropractors who have successfully passed such examinations which include requirements of character and ethics, and providing for the penalization of chiropractors who fail to comply with the provisions of the chiropractic legislation. Penalties may range from censure and suspension through revocation of license, to fine and/or imprisonment.

Of the states that regulate chiropractic, all require at least a high school education as a preliminary requisite to chiropractic education. Many states require chiropractors to have at least two years of liberal-arts college in addition to high school.

All but two of the states regulating chiropractic require that the candidate for a chiropractic license successfully complete a four-year chiropractic course.

Similar requirements prevail in foreign countries. In Canada, six of the seven provinces regulating chiropractic require a junior matriculation certificate or its equivalent—the equal of our high school diploma. Also in these six provinces, successful completion of a four-year chiropractic course is necessary in order to qualify for a license.

Chiropractic's physical plant, too, has grown up over the decades. Although they are fewer in number than the medical institutions, for the simple reason that chiropractic has fewer practitioners and patients, the top-rank chiropractic schools, hospitals, clinics, and mental institutions are rapidly achieving a par in their respective healing field.

CHAPTER EIGHT

X-ray and Chiropractic

As has been pointed out, chiropractic was discovered in 1895, the same year that Prof. Wilhelm Roentgen of Wurzburg, Germany, discovered the X-ray, which was destined to play an important role in the growth and development of the science of chiropractic.

X-rays were so named by Prof. Roentgen because they were then rays of unknown origin which, although they could not be seen, could penetrate the human body and many other substances. X-rays have become invaluable in the healing arts, in industry, and in scientific research.

Since the study of anatomical disrelation, particularly of the bones of the spinal column, is the special province of the chiropractors, it was natural that they should have been among the first professionals to use the X-ray for spinal studies. Even before World War I, in 1910, at a time when glass plates served the purpose for which photographic film is now used, courses in X-ray were given at The Palmer School of Chiropractic in Davenport, Iowa.

During World War I, rapid progress was made in the development of X-ray equipment and techniques.

All the resources of the United States government were directed toward improvements resulting from the discoveries that grew out of the demands made during the European conflict. Films gradually replaced the glass plates that had been used for many years. Film sizes increased, and improved X-ray tubes that could accommodate increased voltage were also produced. Contrast safety films, processed in improved chemicals, all contributed to a better finished product.

By 1918, the Universal College of Chiropractic in Pittsburgh, Pennsylvania, had produced the first X-ray views of the spine taken in the upright position in order to observe the effects of unequal leg lengths, pelvic distortion, and body stress under the influence of gravity. In 1932, Dr. Warren L. Sausser, a chiropractor of New York, produced the first full-length single-exposure X-ray view of the entire spine on a 14 x 36 inch film. This remarkable development enabled an engineering analysis for body distortion in the upright position. It was reported in the *Journal of Radiography and Clinical Photography,* published by the Eastman Kodak Company of Rochester, New York, in the August, 1937 issue (Vol. 13, No. 2).

After considerable experimentation, Dr. Warren Sausser, in 1934, for the first time successfully made a full-body X-ray picture showing the entire skeletal system of an adult human. The Eastman Kodak Company cooperated fully on this project, making a special 20 x 70 inch film. The entire technique for the full-skeleton exposure was described in the February, 1935 issue of the *National Chiropractic Journal.*

In 1940, Dr. Theodore Vladeff, a chiropractor of Detroit, Michigan, invented new apparatus relating to

X-ray processes and improved the means for taking spinal X-ray pictures and for recording the conditions under which such pictures were taken. The process and apparatus were filed with the U.S. Patent Office on April 16, 1940, and the patent was granted August 18, 1942 (U.S. Patent No. 2,293,324). In March, 1953, Dr. Vladeff patented a screen for the control of X-ray exposures. (U.S. Patent No. 2,630,536.) This was filed on November 16, 1949.

Dr. Ernest A. Fox, a chiropractor of Battle Creek, Michigan, filed a patent on June 26, 1953, for an apparatus which would X-ray the spinal column laterally (from the side) and was subsequently granted his patent on December 18, 1956 (U.S. Patent No. 2,774,884).

Stereoscopic X-ray studies of the upper cervical region, developed at The Palmer School of Chiropractic, and X-ray research of the human pelvis by Dr. F. W. Illi, a chiropractor of Geneva, Switzerland, have excited the admiration of European medical researchers, particularly in Switzerland, England, and Germany. Dr. Albert Cramer, a Hamburg physician, and Professor Zuckschwerdt, state in two books on this subject that these studies by Dr. Illi surpass in refinement and precision anything to be found in the entire literature of medicine.

For more than half a century, instruction in the taking of X-ray pictures of the spine and their interpretation has been a standard part of the chiropractic curriculum in every school of chiropractic, and this instruction today consists of 300 class hours and is both theoretical and practical. The subject matter is regarded as an integral part of chiropractic, and research in this field continues to be active among chiropractors on both sides of the Atlantic.

Despite the demonstrated fact that members of the chiropractic profession have been the pioneers of spinal roentgenology, organized medicine continues to attack the competency of doctors of chiropractic in the use of X-ray for diagnostic purposes.

But the scientists and the courts have decided otherwise. There is an erroneous impression that only a licensed medical doctor may be competent to testify as to the taking of X-rays and their interpretation.

Our courts have generally held to the contrary. The mere licensing of a physician does not in itself give him the necessary qualifications. He must first show experience in the taking of X-rays and in their interpretation. The courts have likewise held that it is not necessary that the witness be a member of the medical profession in order to qualify in the interpretation of X-ray plates. The witness must show knowledge of the human anatomy and experience in taking X-ray plates. This problem arose in the case of *Ladlie v. American Glycerine Co., 115 Kan. 507,* where testimony as to the nature of the X-ray plates was given by a chiropractor. The court overruled the objection to his testimony and held:

". . . surely a man who had made a professional study of the human spine, and who had worked with an X-ray for eighteen months, and who had taken 500 or 600 X-ray pictures of parts of the human skeleton, could not be totally disqualified to testify; and any want of thoroughness of his information would only lessen the convincing force of his testimony: it would not bar its consideration altogether."

The amount of experience the witness has may affect the weight of his testimony, but would not be any basis for excluding it.

The court, in *Whipple v. Grandchamp, 261 Mass. 40,* likewise noted that a person, not licensed as a doctor of medicine, who otherwise is experienced in taking and interpreting X-rays, is permitted to testify:

"It is plain that knowledge of the human anatomy may be acquired to a high degree by a student of that subject, although such a person is neither licensed nor registered as a doctor of medicine; and it is equally clear, as a matter of common knowledge, that, in many professions other than medicine, the use of the X-ray is familiar, and that it is read in connection with the human anatomy."

As the courts throughout the country have observed, the X-ray is a scientific and mechanical appliance which may be used by any person schooled in the art and having the requisite scientific knowledge of its properties, and "there would seem to be no reason why its application to the human body may not be explained by any person who understands it," *Henslin v. Wheaton, 91 Minn. 219.*

The X-ray plays an important part in the practice of chiropractic. It determines the condition of the bones of the human framework and the exact position of the spinal misalignment or subluxation. This knowledge is important in that it provides information that will lead to corrective measures.

Surveys made by radiation physicists throughout the country, indicate that radiation hazards in chiropractic offices are kept to a minimum in accord with generally accepted radiographic standards. Professor Edgar N. Grisewood, Director of the Department of Physics, New York University, made such a survey in New York State and reported that in chiropractic offices examined by him at random he found that the doctors of chiropractic employ all the accepted safeguards necessary to minimize exposure.

In 1956, exaggerated fears were raised in the public's mind by blowing up a scare smoke screen about "atomic radiation" with reference to the taking of X-rays for health purposes. In 1961, a sober reappraisal of the situation began, according to William C. Stronach, Executive Secretary of the American College of Radiology. This has been brought about by an educational program for all who use X-ray equipment. The chiropractic profession has been in the forefront in this program with the establishment of "Radiation Commissions" created by its national organizations.

It is now recognized that X-rays are essential in the diagnosis of a wide range of disorders, and that a patient who refuses to be X-rayed because of fear of radiation would not be protecting his health but jeopardizing it.

Part Two

RESULTS ACHIEVED
BY CHIROPRACTIC

CHAPTER NINE

Seeking the Source of Good Health

Evidence of increasing interest in and acceptance of chiropractic is the recent invitation by the *University of Toronto Medical Journal* to Dr. A. G. Homewood, Dean of the Canadian Memorial Chiropractic College, Toronto, to write an article for the *Medical Journal* which would clarify the position of chiropractic in the healing arts.

Dr. Homewood submitted a detailed article, published in the February, 1961 issue of the *University of Toronto Medical Journal,* which describes the progress of the profession and presents an explanation of the role of chiropractic in health and disease. He states in part:

"The doctor of chiropractic must have an efficient working knowledge of the distribution of the nerve fibres for both diagnostic and treatment purposes, since his entire concept hinges upon the importance of the nervous system in the control of function in both health and disease. The patient is examined with a view to determining not only the named symptom complex but also the structural disrelation causing the disturbance to the nervous system with the subsequent alterations in function and tissue changes of pathology. Here lies the basic difference between the practice of allopathic medicine and chiropractic. The allopathic practitioner will concern himself with prescribing a drug to counteract the associated microorganisms, stimulate the function retarded, or inhibit the function exhibiting excess. The chiropractor would attempt to adjust the structure to remove interference with normal nerve transmission, in the expectation that the body alone has the innate knowledge of how to heal and restore normal function. He is not concerned, therefore, with attempting to stimulate or inhibit, but rather, he seeks to normalize. To do a thorough service for his patient, the chiropractor should attempt to determine the background cause of the structural distortion and have such cause, or causes, eradicated. The chiropractor appreciates that not every case will respond to his particular approach and that there are those cases that must be referred to the surgeon, the dentist, oculist, etc. Furthermore, there may be a need to utilize antibiotics in some cases of infection, insulin for the diabetic, morphine for severe pain; in such cases, the allopathic physician is called and the patient referred. The chiropractor is very conscious of the fact that he does not have the panacea for all ills.

"While the chiropractor has earned particular recognition in the field of somatic disorders, such as the lumbar-spinal problems, neuritis, sciatica, etc., ever increasing numbers of the population are appreciating the fact that the chiropractor has a general health service to render that is efficacious in the greater percentage of conditions. Therefore, many families depend upon him for care of all conditions, leaving the decision as to when to consult other members of the healing arts to his judgment. Expectant mothers and obstetricians are often surprised at the ease with which delivery is effected when the mother has received chiropractic care during the pregnancy—making the necessary corrections incidental to the stress of unusual weight distribution, assuring proper elimination, and nutritional intake. Children respond readily to the techniques of the chiropractor and are guarded against the ill effects of structural distortion occasioned by falls, as well as being guided in the development of correct posture. Chiropractic is concerned with the patient who has the disease, rather than the disease that has the patient. In other words, if assistance is given to a sick body and it has the power within itself to effect healing, chiropractic can be effective. In the event that the pathology is irreversible, or the patient does not have the vitality to respond, then surgery or other methods may be necessitated. Some of the claims being made for the effectiveness of chiropractic by German and other European medical doctors would make the average chiropractor blush. Many of these investigators have been quoted in a recently published book, *Medicine and Chiropractic* by C. W. Weiant and S. Goldschmidt."

Here is an example which shows the chiropractic approach to a health problem.

Let us suppose you are crossing the street and suddenly have to jump out of the way of an oncoming truck that has just come around the corner. In the process of saving your life, you may twist your entire body. You feel a slight twinge of pain, but nothing more; and you think nothing more about it.

However, that twist of your body may have caused a sufficient distortion of your spine to affect very seriously one or more nerve channels emanating from the spinal column. The resultant interference with the normal flow of nervous energy will ultimately cause symptoms of one sort or another—depending on which nerves were affected and which organs they supply.

Generally, the first symptoms will be felt immediately—neuritis, stiff neck, backache, laryngitis, stomach pains; any one of a number of conditions could be triggered off. Numerous disease patterns are always within our bodies only awaiting the encouragement of a disturbed body structure and an impeded nervous system to develop into activity. Some of them become apparent immediately, others may take weeks or months to develop, possibly, into serious conditions.

When the first symptom appears, the chiropractor seeks the cause behind it. He wants above all to restore natural harmony between the structures of the body, and to bring the nervous system back to its proper functioning.

In doing this job, by means of spinal adjustment and other corrective measures, the chiropractor will of course be correcting the symptoms which have already appeared. But he is doing more than that. He cannot avoid doing more, because of the very nature of his approach.

In the process of restoring the body to a well-functioning state, the chiropractor is preventing the outbreak of symptoms for which the foundations may already have been laid, but which have not yet developed. In putting the body back in shape to fight off the symptoms of the backache, or the neuritis, or the stiff neck, or the head cold, the chiropractor automatically, and at the same time, puts the body in shape to prevent other ailments which are still in process of maturing.

Preventing a recurrence of the symptom is, for the chiropractor, the first step. At the same time, he is treating the entire body. The net result will be that the person will have a better-functioning nervous system and an improvement in structural balance.

These, combined with sound hygienic habits and good nutrition will lead to greater efficiency and greater health.

In this sense, the chiropractor is a "doctor of health" rather than a "disease treater." He serves a most important function in this modern world where the hazards of daily living put strains on us that make the preservation of health more important than ever before.

A good part of "organized medicine" has waged a strong and persistent attack on chiropractic—a political and economic war in which numerous M.D.'s do not really wish to participate. In view of the "official" thumbs-down on chiropractic by the medical organization, it seems important to examine some of the results that have been claimed for chiropractic in terms of personal case histories.

First, however, let us quote at some length from a recent study written by a medical doctor, Charles Greenberg, M.D., and entitled *Report on Spinal Adjustment and Its Relationship to Health and Disease.* Since this report is by a medical man who prepared it for the medical profession, it cannot be considered as biased in favor of chiropractic. Secondly, it contains a comprehensive summary of the ailments chiropractic has helped. Thus, it may be considered a rough outline of the case for chiropractic in terms of results achieved. Dr. Greenberg writes:

"Time and again this theory (the chiropractic theory of spinal adjustment) has been confirmed, not only by chiropractic but by eminent leaders of medical science.

"The following conditions are the ones which respond successfully and quickly to spinal adjustments:

"Sacro-iliac strain, neuralgias of arms, legs, back, and face.

"Neuritis and sciatica.

"Asthma.

"Migraine, and all other types of severe headaches; dizziness, nervous tension.

"Lumbago, and all other back pains.

"The above respond with dramatic results with as few as three to four treatments.

"These are the conditions which give the greatest amount of successful results (not just temporary relief) with spinal adjustments.

"Many other conditions, too numerous to mention, are also greatly helped when other types of medical treatments fail.

". . . many members of the medical profession have spoken up vigorously at one time or another in support of the principles of chiropractic. Sometimes it is because they have observed the remarkable results achieved by chiropractic after medical methods have failed. At other times, it results from scientific investigations which reveal that chiropractic has indeed something to offer those seeking health."

Dr. Greenberg then quotes a number of medical authorities, including B. Gomroe of the University of Pennsylvania Medical School, who observed in his recent book, *Arthritis and Allied Conditions:* "In a group of patients with low-back pains . . . these respond well to manipulative (chiropractic) measures. It is this type of patient who may be 'miraculously cured' by certain mechanical maneuvers of chiropractors which are frowned upon and looked askance on by the medical profession. If physicians realized that manipulative procedures properly performed may produce a good result in some conditions, the great mass of these patients would not resort to cults other than orthodox medicine."

Chiropractors, of course, object strenuously to being classified as members of a "cult" or as "cultists." They say that their studies of the nervous system, of the spine, and of spinal adjustment are just as scientific and thorough as anything undertaken by medical men.

The ailments discussed in what follows here are grouped according to regions of the body. General categories of sickness are grouped into miscellaneous ills, children's ailments, and mental ailments. The breakdown is as simple as possible, covering the upper portion of the body down to the diaphragm, and the remainder of the body below the diaphragm. The remainder of Part Two, consequently, is divided into five chapters, detailing the benefits of chiropractic:

(a) in head and upper-body ills;

(b) in visceral and lower-body ills, including "low-back" conditions;

(c) in general ills;

(d) in children's ailments;

(e) in mental ailments.

CHAPTER TEN

Chiropractic in Head and Upper-Body Ills

The information in this and the next four chapters comes from case records of chiropractic patients and statistical surveys. Some of the details have been taken from newspaper accounts; most of them are from the records of chiropractors in various parts of the country. The case records are based on the statements of the patients themselves. Chiropractic associations and clinics have recently undertaken the compilation of field-research studies of cases given chiropractic care. Selections of survey material from two of the most recent and continuing field studies are also included in the following pages.

1. **Allergy:** Field Survey Data
   Number of cases: 39   Male: 19   Female: 20
   Average age: 23.5 years
       Youngest: 1 year   Oldest: 70 years
   Duration of condition: Average—7.4 years
                          Longest—25 years
                          Shortest—60 days

Length of chiropractic care:
   Average—140.5 days
Number having previous chiropractic care: 7
   Medical: 33

Summary	Number	%
Recovered	22	56.4
Much improved	12	30.8
Some improvement	4	10.3
No improvement	1	2.5
Worse	0	0

2. Amnesia:

The following is quoted verbatim from the *Phoenix* (Arizona) *Republic* of April 30, 1953:

"Phoenix police did what they always did with amnesia victims yesterday and, sure enough, the victim remembered everything.

"In the middle of the afternoon a man came into the station. He was crying. He told Sgt. Arthur Fairbanks the past was a blank. The man said the last he remembered was being on a bus from Tucson to Phoenix.

"Fairbanks went into a huddle with Capt. Morehead. 'Take him to Dr. Shelton,' Morehead said.

"The Captain was speaking of Dr. Milburn C. Shelton, Glendale chiropractor, who police say has restored 19 memories in a row.

"Patrolman Norman Morris and Leonard Damiani watched as the doctor manipulated the vertebrae in the victim's neck.

" 'He went to sleep for a few minutes,' Norris said.

102

'Then he woke up, looked at our uniforms, and wanted to know if he had done anything wrong.'

"The man remembered he was Hugh E. Smith of Covina, California. He remembered he was 40 years old, had a wife, and five children. It all came back to him, he said, that he went to Tucson last Sunday to look for work."

3. Asthma: R.A., a young man of 22, had suffered from asthma since the age of eight. The frequent choking attacks made it difficult for him to work or associate with friends. He received treatment at the Asthma Clinic of the New York Hospital and had had injections which gave some relief, although the attacks always recurred. He was advised to avoid dust, feather pillows, rugs, and tobacco smoke. He finally went to a chiropractor. X ray revealed displacements of the second and third dorsal vertebrae. He was adjusted three times per week. After the first week of adjustments his condition improved markedly, and in three months he recovered completely.

4. Asthma: Field Survey Data
   Number of cases: 355 Male: 188 Female: 167
   Average age: 32.9 years   Youngest: 1 year
                                  Oldest: 79 years
   Duration of condition: Average—9.7 years
                             Longest—57 years
                             Shortest—7 days
   Length of chiropractic care:
      Average—117.9 days
   Number having previous chiropractic care: 71
    Medical: 340

Summary	Number	%
Recovered	146	41.1
Much improved	140	39.4
Some improvement	43	12.1
No improvement	23	6.5
Worse	3	.9

5. **Hay Fever:** Field Survey Data
Number of cases: 141 **Male:** 75 **Female:** 66
Average age: 30.7 years
    Youngest: 4 years.   Oldest: 72 years
Duration of condition: Average—10 years
                           Longest—50 years
                           Shortest—7 days
Length of chiropractic care:
    Average—111 days
Number having previous chiropractic care: 32
    Medical: 130

Summary	Number	%
Recovered	65	46.1
Much improved	50	35.5
Some improvement	19	13.4
No improvement	7	5.0
Worse	0	0

6. **Headache:** Following an accident in which he was "badly shaken up," C.D. of Roseau, Minnesota, had severe headaches which sometimes lasted for several days and were almost unendurable. Over a period of years, he underwent treatment by several medical doctors, but nothing they did helped for "more than a short time." He then went to a chiro-

practor, who X-rayed his neck and stated that the first bone in the spine, just below the head, was slightly out of place. One adjustment greatly improved the condition. The patient visits the chiropractor infrequently, since he lives 150 miles distant, but writes that he's "free of headaches for weeks at a time and they are never very severe, now."

7. **Headache:** Clinic Statistics
   Number of cases: 145 Male: 33 Female: 112
   Average age: 36.4 years
       Youngest: 6 years   Oldest: 71 years
   Duration of condition: Average—7.9 years
                              Longest—35 years
                              Shortest—2 weeks
   Length of chiropractic care:
       Average—2.4 months
   Number having previous chiropractic care: 27
       Medical: 69

Summary	Number	%
Recovered	54	37.3
Much improved	46	31.7
Some improvement	25	17.3
No improvement	20	13.7
Worse	0	0

8. **Hiccoughs:** V.T. of Hot Springs, Arkansas, had a severe attack of hiccoughs which lasted for over three weeks. Five medical doctors attended the patient at various times, but "no permanent relief" resulted. Then the patient visited a chiropractor, and two adjustments were given, the first at 11:30 A.M. and the sec-

ond at 1:15 P.M. Shortly after the second adjustment, the hiccoughs ceased and did not return thereafter.

9. **Meniere's Disease:** Field Survey Data
   Number of cases: 25 Male: 16 Female: 9
   Average age: 51 years
      Youngest: 21 years   Oldest: 71 years
   Duration of condition: Average—5.3 years
                            Longest—15 years
                            Shortest—7 days
   Length of chiropractic care:
      Average—131.8 days
   Number having previous chiropractic care: 3
      Medical: 21

Summary	Number	%
Recovered	10	40.0
Much improved	8	32.0
Some improvement	5	20.0
No improvement	2	8.0
Worse	0	0

10. **Sinusitis:** For twelve years, Mrs. A.O.S. of Dayton, Ohio, suffered with a severe sinus condition which produced headaches so painful that frequently she could not lie down but had to sit up and hold her head in her hands. Treatment by numerous medical doctors did no good, and the patient was advised to move to a drier climate. At that point she visited a chiropractor, and after three adjustments the headaches vanished for the first time in two years. After four months, the patient was so much improved that her headaches virtually ceased and she discontinued wearing heavily tinted glasses.

11. **Chronic Sinusitis:** Field Survey Data
    Number of cases: 423 **Male:** 231 **Female:** 192
    Average age: 39.9 years
       Youngest: 4 years   Oldest: 80 years
    Duration of condition: Average—8.8 years
                              Longest—53 years
                              Shortest—5 days
    Length of chiropractic care:
       Average—93.5 days
    Number having previous chiropractic care: 116
       Medical: 383

Summary	Number	%
Recovered	173	40.9
Much improved	179	42.3
Some improvement	50	11.8
No improvement	20	4.7
Worse	1	.3

12. **Torticollis:** Field Survey Data
    Number of cases: 208 **Male:** 124 **Female:** 84
    Average age: 37 years
       Youngest: 4 years Oldest: 78 years
    Duration of condition: Average—6.9 years
                              Longest—50 years
                              Shortest—1 day
    Length of chiropractic care:
       Average—24.1 days
    Number having previous chiropractic care: 56
       Medical: 111

Summary	Number	%
Recovered	154	74.0
Much improved	40	19.2

Some improvement	9	4.4
No improvement	5	2.4
Worse	0	0

CHAPTER ELEVEN

Chiropractic in Visceral and Lower-Body Ills, Including "Low-Back" Conditions

The following dramatic story is condensed from *The Houston* (Texas) *Post* of February 28, 1949:

While working in a shipyard during World War II, Robert Harold Harmon was struck in the back by a section of steel bulkhead. It knocked his spine out of line as thoroughly as a right-angle collision would distort the frame of an automobile that was struck from the side.

". . . some of the best Houston medical men in one of the leading hospitals told him that he would never be able to lift more than 25 pounds." Harmon himself said, ". . . they told me I was one-hundred per cent disabled, a cripple for the rest of my life."

Harmon's back, from his shoulders to the base of his spine, was fitted with "cumbersome braces and irksome supports" which gave him "only slight help." He believed himself doomed "to totter through life, pain-wracked and bitter."

Then the medical doctors made a final suggestion. According to Harmon: "They wanted to lay my back wide open. 'You may or may not improve,' they said."

Friends advised Harmon to try a chiropractor. This

was in 1948. Harmon didn't think much of the idea: "I never had any faith in chiropractors," he said.

But he went to a chiropractor, just the same. The man took several X rays and told Harmon that "practically the entire length of his back was misaligned." He began adjustments.

"Within two weeks' time I was able to discard the brace," Harmon said in 1949. "Within two months, I was practically healed and I have never worn the brace since then. I still have minor pains, but I believe if I had gone to a chiropractor in the beginning, I would be without any difficulty today." He bent his better than six-foot height and easily touched his finger tips to the floor. "I can tackle anything from a cup to a refrigerator," he said. "I told that chiropractor that he'd have to prove it to me—he did!"

Low-Back Syndrome (complex of symptoms): In the latter part of 1947, the Research Council of the New York State Chiropractic Society undertook a survey of the problem of low-back pain. Data sought included age, sex, occupation, location of patient's pain, etiology, previous diagnosis and treatment, chiropractic analysis, number of adjustments, and the length of time under chiropractic care.

Four hundred and eighty-one cases were reported. Of these, 327 were males and 154 females. Their occupations included plumber, electrician, mechanic, carpenter, machinist, mason, painter, plasterer, upholsterer, housewife, tailor, boilermaker, brewer, welder, and other classifications where occupational hazards are great. There were a few professional persons such as accountants, architects, clergymen, pharmacists, physicians, teachers, attorneys, and dentists.

The average number of adjustments required per patient was 10.5, with 47 patients requiring only one adjustment and one requiring 160. Three hundred and forty-nine of the patients (72 per cent) recovered completely under chiropractic, 100 or 21 per cent showed improvement, while only 32 or seven per cent showed no improvement. (Source: The *New York State Chiropractic Journal,* December, 1948. X rays of the above-mentioned patients before and after treatment are available.)

Following are some of the case histories:

E.G. Female, age 38, housewife. Experienced frequent attacks of right-sided sciatica over a period of 10 years, apparently caused by a severe fall. Previous care: medical and osteopathic. Patient had been bedridden for three months at the time the chiropractor was consulted. X-rays were taken and revealed a right sacroiliac slip, with pronounced body distortion toward the head. In one month, after 12 adjustments, the patient was symptom free.

W.F. Male, age 34, clerical worker. Upon arising one morning, was seized with acute low-back pain. The symptoms seemed to increase in severity until the patient was so completely incapacitated that he was unable to work for a period of six months. A number of physicians were consulted, each one attempting a different mode of treatment, but with negligible results. X-rays taken by a chiropractor revealed compensatory scoliosis with a pronounced pelvic list and antero-inferiority of the sacrum. After two weeks of daily adjustment, the patient was completely relieved, whereupon he resumed his occupation. He received 15 adjustments in all within 21 days. When the chiropractor saw the patient some two years later, the latter reported that there had been no recurrence of either pain or disability.

M.S. Male, age 41, certified public accountant. Experienced acute left sciatic pain following trauma encountered while doing physical exercises. Physician was consulted, and lower back was strapped with adhesive. After several weeks of pain, the patient consulted an orthopedic surgeon and was hospitalized. A plaster cast was applied for a period of 17 days, followed by daily diathermy routine. The sciatic pain seemed to persist, and the discouraged patient asked for discharge from the hospital. A chiropractor was consulted. Initial roentgenograms in the upright position showed a badly tipped pelvis with a right leg deficiency of three-fourths of an inch. Patient was completely symptom free after two months of chiropractic (adjustments daily).

H.S. Male, age 52, a surgeon. Referred to a chiropractor by a colleague. Gave a history of intermittent attacks of low-back disability ranging over a period of 14 years. Etiology was uncertain. Routine orthopedic care and and physiotherapy had given no relief.

The patient complained of severe pain radiating into the left groin and was unable to stand erect, evidencing marked muscle spasm in the left erector group. X-rays revealed a left rotatory scoliosis, asymmetry of the lumbo-sacral facets, right pelvic sway, and a slight lipping of the bodies of the fourth and fifth lumbar bodies. The patient was adjusted daily for eight days and was completely free from pain at the end of that period. He was able to resume his occupation after the third adjustment. During three succeeding years, there was one slight recurrence, which was corrected by a single adjustment.

The 42 chiropractors who reported in this survey stated that when cases were detected involving actual disease of the bones, spinal-cord tumors, malignancies, and degenerative diseases of bone and adjacent structures, the patients were referred to medical doctors and orthopedic surgeons. "The services of the neurosurgeon, orthopedic surgeon, podiatrist, and other specialists are oft times indicated," the report noted. This would seem to give the lie to charges that chiropractors attempt to "cure everything."

Herniated Disc: (slipped disc) Field Survey Data
Number of cases: 1030 Male: 772 Female: 258
Average age: 32.6 years
   Youngest: 15 years   Oldest: 86 years
Duration of condition: Average—4.5 years
                             Longest—50 years
                             Shortest—1 day
Length of chiropractic care:
   Average—76.4 days
Number having previous chiropractic care: 280
   Medical: 858

Summary	Number	%
Recovered	513	49.8
Much improved	396	38.4
Some improvement	81	7.9

No improvement   36   3.5

Worse   4   .4

Total number well or some improvement—990
of Total—96.1%

Lumbago: Field Survey Data
Number of cases: 1835
  Male: 1204   Female: 631
Average age: 40.7 years
  Youngest: 9 years   Oldest: 79 years
Duration of condition: Average—6.5 years
                          Longest—54 years
                          Shortest—1 day
Length of chiropractic care:
  Average—67.2 days
Number having previous chiropractic care: 475
  Medical: 1358

Summary	Number	%
Recovered	983	53.6
Much improved	619	33.7
Some improvement	147	8.0
No improvement	76	4.2
Worse	10	.5

Total number well or some improvement—1749
of Total—95.3%

Research has verified the viscero-spinal principle
that nerve irritation at the spine may lead to a disturbance of one or more internal organs of the body. This
explains the effectiveness of chiropractic in dealing
with the following conditions:

Gall-Bladder Disturbance: Mrs. M. K. of Ontario,

Canada, suffered from a gall-bladder condition (so diagnosed by medical doctors) for 35 years. She experienced "terrible pains" in the "intestinal region," under the shoulder, and through the back. Numerous medical doctors succeeded in giving her only "temporary relief." Then she went to a chiropractor, although she wondered how he could help her "without medicine or another operation." After three months of adjustment she felt "like a new woman."

Menstrual Disorders: Field Survey Data
Number of cases: 269
Average age: 29.9 years
   Youngest: 12 years   Oldest: 59 years
Duration of condition: Average—6.6 years
                             Longest—30 years
                             Shortest—3 days
Length of chiropractic care:
   Average—98.2 days
Number having previous chiropractic care: 51
   Medical: 241

Summary	Number	%
Recovered	107	39.8
Much improved	113	42.0
Some improvement	32	11.9
No improvement	16	5.9
Worse	1	.4

Total number well or some improvement—252
   of Total—93.7%

Stomach Trouble and Nervousness: For eight years, A. J. D. of Loveland, Ohio, had suffered acutely;

despite medical treatment he was "getting worse all the time." He wrote: "I had consulted eight different medical doctors, besides going through the clinic of the largest hospital in this part of the country. All the tests and all the diagnoses and all the prescriptions and all the 'shots' and all the drugs and all the treatments did not help me." At this point he went to a chiropractor. In "about six months" his ailments were "completely corrected."

Stomach Ulcers: J. L. of Salt Lake City, Utah, was under medical care for ulcers of the stomach "off and on for 10 years." The various medicines and diets prescribed sometimes brought temporary relief. Most of the medical doctors this patient visited recommended surgery. He finally went to a chiropractor, and subsequently wrote: "Shortly after I began taking adjustments, I was delighted to find that I could eat all kinds of food without distress and could forget about diets."

Stomach Ulcers: Field Survey Data
Number of cases: 167 Male: 134 Female: 33
Average age: 44.4 years
   Youngest: 16 years   Oldest: 79 years
Duration of condition: Average—7.3 years
                           Longest—36 years
                           Shortest—8 days
Length of chiropractic care:
   Average—122.1 days
Number having previous chiropractic care: 32
   Medical: 161

Summary	Number	%
Recovered	62	37.1
Much improved	72	43.1
Some improvement	22	13.2
No improvement	10	6.0
Worse	1	.6

Total number well or some improvement—156
of Total—93.4%

CHAPTER TWELVE

Chiropractic in General Ills

Following are a few of the many documented cases and research studies of chiropractic results in dealing with general ills of the body:

Arthritis: Mrs. A. S. of Glendale, New York, had arthritis and accompanying serious bone deformities in her feet, wrists, and hands. For about 15 years, she underwent various medical treatments, including medications, vaccines, heat treatments, and removal of the tonsils with an electric needle. "The only change in my condition was for the worse," the patient wrote. Chiropractic was then suggested to her, and after two years of adjustments, she wrote that she was once again "able to enjoy life, free from the discomforts of arthritic pain and in greatly improved general health."

Arthritis: Mrs. J. W. P. of Ft. Valley, Georgia, wrote: "For fourteen months I suffered with arthritis and was treated by a number of medical doctors in different hospitals. At one time I lay on a board for four weeks, had my tonsils removed, was given all kinds of intravenous and muscular shots, and took enough medicine to fill a drug store. All of this gave absolutely no relief and I determined to try chiropractic as a last resort." After two months of adjustments, she was "practically well."

Arthritis (rheumatoid): J. T. S. of Brooklyn, New York, was unable to raise his arms and could not even reach his face. He wrote: "I had no appetite—food nauseated me. My neck was stiff, my left knee swollen. My back was stiff and I could not bend to put my shoes on. My arms, legs, ankles, and hands pained, and I had no strength left in my hands at all—I couldn't even tie a string." He went to various medical doctors and to a hospital without benefit; after a week of hospital examination, he was told that nothing could be done for him. At this point a friend recommended a chiropractor. He wrote after a little less than four months of adjustments: "Today, while not completely cured, I can get around by myself without help and little or no pain."

Arthritis: Field Survey Data
Number of cases: 447   Male: 197   Female: 250
Average age: 51 years
 Youngest: 5 years   Oldest: 79 years
Duration of condition: Average—8.5 years
  Longest—27 years
  Shortest—21 days
Length of chiropractic care:
 Average—111.7 days
Number having previous chiropractic care: 105
Medical: 412

Summary	Number	%
Recovered	111	24.8

Much improved	217	48.5
Some improvement	75	16.8
No improvement	42	9.4
Worse	2	.5

Total number well or some improvement—403 of Total—90.1%

Common Cold: A. R. of Bellmore, Long Island, suffered "continuously" from colds for at least seven years. Medical doctors prescribed the "usual medicines and nose drops." A tonsillectomy was advised. Not wanting the operation, the patient went to a chiropractor. She received adjustment for "about three months, at an average of two to three adjustments a week." Her tonsils became healthy and her colds cleared up; after five years, she reported "splendid health."

Acute and Chronic Colds: Field Survey Data
Number of cases: 272 Male: 145 Female: 127
Average age: 31.9 years
   Youngest: 1 year   Oldest: 79 years
Duration of condition: Average—8.1 years
                             Longest—50 years
                             Shortest—2 days
Length of chiropractic care:
   Average—68.3 days
Number having previous chiropractic care: 45
   Medical: 197

Summary	Number	%
Recovered	156	57.4
Much improved	88	32.4
Some improved	17	6.2

No improvement	11	4.0
Worse	0	0

Total number well or some improvement—261
  of Total—96%

Eczema (chronic): J. K. of Coronado suffered from severe eczema for more than 10 years. She tried everything she could think of for it—"medical doctors, skin specialists, and every kind of doctor anyone suggested." Nothing helped. Her appearance was so bad that she lost one position after another and finally had to stop working altogether. She itched constantly. Then chiropractic was suggested; she went to a chiropractor, and after a few months wrote: "Besides my skin clearing up, my general health has improved."

Eczema: Field Survey Data
Number of cases: 52 Male: 23 Female: 29
Average age: 26.2 years
  Youngest: 1 year   Oldest: 69 years
Duration of condition: Average—6.8 years
                          Longest—30 years
                          Shortest—14 days
Length of chiropractic care:
  Average—110 days
Number having previous chiropractic care: 12
  Medical: 48

Summary	Number	%
Recovered	29	55.8
Much improved	15	28.8
Some improvement	3	5.8
No improvement	5	9.6
Worse	0	0

Total number well or some improvement—47
of Total—93.4%

Hypertension: N. K. of New York City suffered for over 10 years with blood pressure ratings
varying from 230 to 240. He was under the care of a
prominent medical heart specialist for the last two
years, but there was no improvement. The specialist
said the condition was caused by lesions in the heart
and aorta. After one month of chiropractic adjustments, the blood pressure had dropped to 200; at
the end of three months, it was 170. After eight
months, the patient was discharged with blood pressure maintained between 160 and 170.

Hypertension: Field Survey Data
Number of cases: 316 Male: 116 Female: 200
Average age: 54.4 years
    Youngest: 19 years   Oldest: 89 years
Duration of condition: Average—7.8 years
                          Longest—30 years
                          Shortest—2 days
Length of chiropractic care:
    Average—96 days
Number having previous chiropractic care: 66
    Medical: 287

Summary	Number	%
Recovered	86	27.2
Much improved	145	45.8
Some improvement	61	19.3
No improvement	20	6.4
Worse	4	1.3

Total number well or some improvement—292
  of Total—92.3%

Hypotension: Field Survey Data
Number of cases: 91 Male: 47 Female: 44
Average age: 42.2 years
  Youngest: 19 years   Oldest: 72 years
Duration of condition: Average—8.5 years
                      Longest—23 years
                      Shortest—3 days
Length of chiropractic care:
  Average—95.4 days
Number having previous chiropractic care: 16
  Medical: 76

Summary	Number	%
Recovered	28	30.8
Much improved	39	42.8
Some improvement	16	17.6
No improvement	8	8.8
Worse	0	0

Total number well or some improvement—83
  of Total—91.2%

123

CHAPTER THIRTEEN

Chiropractic in Children's Ailments

The following is quoted verbatim from the *Atlanta* (Ga.) *Constitution:*

"The stone mask that four years ago crept over the lovely features of little Daisy Waller, eight, victim of the rare malady, scleroderma, slowly but surely turning her to stone, today is gone. The lethargy has lifted—leaving no trace.

"The child who once was doomed to death because the tissues of her body were petrifying is playing in her front yard on South Chandler road, apparently the picture of health. She said yesterday: 'I feel good now, just as though I had never been sick. I can play baseball all day long if I want to and ride my bicycle, and I can eat anything I want.'

" 'My teacher sent me home,' she had told her mother, who immediately put the child to bed. For weeks the malady had progressed with alarming speed. She was gradually losing use of her limbs and a strange hardening process of the tissues became apparent to the touch. The muscles began to lose their resiliency.

"After a number of consultations the child's condition was said to be hopeless. Her father and mother, Mr. and Mrs. C. H. Waller, and her six sisters and two brothers watched her condition with a feeling of despair.

"Then the family lawyer recommended an Atlanta chiropractor with the hope that the child could be brought to recovery. Eight weeks after the beginning of the disease, Daisy was X-rayed and treatment was begun. Following the adjustment made three days following the X ray, the child began to respond, and in three weeks a marked change was noted."

The following is quoted verbatim from the *New York Daily Mirror*:

"Four years ago today, Margaret and Thomas Curran brought their ten-month-old son James home from the hospital as a tiny crippled bundle with staring, sightless eyes.

" 'You are lucky he is alive,' the doctors said. 'He'll never see, he'll never talk, he'll never walk.'

"Today, Jimmy will leave his home at 51 North 11th Street, Paterson, New Jersey, and come to New York to see the Armistice Day Parade. He'll walk to the reviewing stand, and, if he is pleased with the soldiers passing by, he'll tell his happy mother all about it.

"This miraculous metamorphosis Mrs. Curran attributes to a special massage Jim has received since the fall of 1938.

"Mrs. Curran told a *Mirror* reporter yesterday

that the baby became ill when they were visiting friends at Pomona, New York, in the summer of 1937. He was taken to Paterson General Hospital, where the malady was diagnosed as bulbar infantile paralysis, a disease survived by one in a thousand. And that one survivor has always been crippled for life.

"After two months, on Armistice Day, Jimmy was taken home. Mrs. Curran brought him to several New York hospitals, where the specialists confirmed the opinion that Jimmy could not be helped and that he would never walk or see.

"Mr. Curran, now a defense worker, and his wife, both begged the doctors to try an operation. They said none would aid the boy.

"The mother engaged a masseur. After the first treatment, the child's stiffened muscles seemed to relax . . .

"In the spring of 1940, the boy made sounds which gradually developed into normal speech. His fingers started to curl, and he found he could pick up things. Then he began to sit up, and one day he pointed a finger at an object and showed he was beginning to see. Two months ago, Jimmy's sight really began to develop, so that now it is completely normal. He still has difficulty on stairs, but the Currans are confident that with continued massage he will be entirely normal soon."

The only trouble with the above story is the use of the words "masseur" and "massage." The practitioner who worked with Jimmy Curran was not a masseur; he was a chiropractor, Dr. M. Kronman of New Jersey.

The Currans were contacted for an explanation. Mrs. Curran confirmed that a chiropractor, and not a masseur, had been working with Jimmy. She added that on September 18, 1937, the baby was taken ill with chills and fever. Hospitalized, his illness was diagnosed as bulbar infantile paralysis; subsequently the condition was rediagnosed as meningitis. Blood transfusions were advised. Finally the baby was sent home. According to a letter written by Mrs. Curran:

". . . his body was cold . . . paralyzed. His head was enlarged, and he was totally blind, of which we knew nothing. No eye doctor had examined him; even Dr. M—— said no eye physician had seen him in his two-months' stay in the hospital.

"We took him to New York Medical Center, but they gave him up as hopeless after two days there. There was nothing they could do.

"They advised me to put him in an institution, have another baby, and try to forget him for my other child's sake. But we kept on trying. We took him to several other hospitals and doctors, but none of them could do any good. He would remain as he was until death . . . Daddy came home from work one day and said he had heard of a good chiropractor he was going to take the baby to . . . I went with him but had given up all hopes for Jimmy, as he had at that time lain as if dead for six months. But to my surprise, after a few treatments, he smiled again. After a few months of treatments, I was so sure his sight was coming back that I took him back to the Medical Center, but they said it was my imagination, that he never would see and that there was not a doctor anywhere who could help him. But we still kept on with the chiropractor and Jimmy kept on improving.

"He is four years old now and can hear, see, speak, and has the intelligence of a five-year-old boy, and in a few months I expect to have him running around, and he will take quite a few steps without help."

In another instance a boy, aged eight, had severe headaches, which often compelled his absence from school over a period of three and one-half years. Then his younger brother wandered away and was temporarily lost. Upon hearing of this, both eyes of the older brother turned in, and the left side of his face became paralyzed.

A medical doctor offered no encouragement. Chiropractic adjustments over a period of 17 days eliminated both the cross-eyed condition and the facial paralysis.

Following are a number of capsule case histories, selected at random:

A baby specialist diagnosed a ten-week-old girl as having a stomach tumor and advised surgical removal if she could be built up sufficiently through blood transfusions to stand the operation. However, the baby worsened and was sent home. At the age of three months, she was "so near death that her stomach and limbs were black from a drying up of the blood in the veins" (parents' letter). After four months of chiropractic adjustments, she was "as active and healthy as any baby could be."

A three-year-old girl developed "St. Vitus' Dance," which generally afflicts children under 15 far more frequently than adults. Medical doctors were unable to help her. She grew worse, her tongue swelled, she could not feed herself or walk, and her speech was impaired. After her first chiropractic adjustment, improvement was noticed, and after two months of adjustments, the condition had completely vanished.

A two-year-old girl gradually developed a whole battery of ailments, including asthma, bronchitis, eczema, bad digestion, and poor elimination. Treatment by at least six different medical doctors produced no benefit. After four months of chiropractic adjustments, "she was entirely well of all her conditions" (mother's letter).

Following a hard fall while jumping rope, a ten-year-old girl developed sleeping sickness. Her parents were told by hospital medical doctors that nothing could be done for her. She was then taken to a chiropractic sanitarium. Within one hour after her first adjustment, she showed improvement, after three days she regained consciousness, and gradually other symptoms such as paralysis of the throat vanished. One month after her first adjustment, "she attended a school picnic, took part in a sixth-grade running race, and won second place . . . Today she is as well and happy as any child could be" (parents' letter).

In November of 1946, a nine-year-old boy was expected to die of asthma before the end of the year. The asthmatic seizures were throttling him a dozen times a day and his heart was weakening. Medical specialists said they could do nothing more for him. A radio appeal by his mother set a dramatic chain of events in motion. Chiropractic was suggested. A U.S. Navy captain flew the boy in his personal plane to St. Louis, and from there he traveled by commercial airline to a Colorado chiropractic sanitarium. He reached the sanitarium on November 6, weighing 50 pounds. On New Year's Day, he weighed 62 pounds and was very much alive, having had only one mild attack of asthma since chiropractic adjustments started.

An unusual case was that of Winifred Gardella who was stricken with polio at the age of three. Winifred was chosen "cover girl" in the March of Dimes campaigns in 1952 and 1953. She was depicted in a hospital crib and was diagnosed as a "helpless paraplegic," sentenced to a life of crutches and braces. After two years of medical treatment, the verdict was "no hope." In 1954, she was put under the care of a doctor of chiropractic, Dr. Lewis Robertson of Santa Cruz, California. After six months of chiropractic care, Winifred Gardella was able to walk without her braces or crutches.

CLINIC STATISTICS

Diagnosis: Poliomyelitis (Chronic)

Number of cases: 11   Male: 5   Female: 6

Average age: 14 years

    Youngest: 4 years   Oldest: 35 years

Duration of condition: Average—3.4 years

                                 Longest—20 years

                                 Shortest—1 week

Length of chiropractic care:

    Average—6.5 months

Number having previous chiropractic care: 2
    Medical: 8

Summary	Number	%
Recovered	2	18.2
Much improved	6	54.6
Some improvement	2	18.2
No improvement	1	9
Worse	0	0

Literally, a multitude of other case histories might be given, but these should be sufficient to indicate that the claims of chiropractic in regard to the handling of children's ills are worth considering. There are many reasons why the spines of the young are subject to strains—even before and at birth—that may cause misalignment. According to Chittenden Turner in *The Rise of Chiropractic*:

"Various abnormalities in children are traceable to impingements on the nerves as affecting cellular activity and predispositions to certain ailments. Adenoids, affections of the ears, nose, and general head disturbances are largely due to the unnecessary force used by persons assisting at birth. Jerking of children by the head frequently causes impingements, and this is given as a cause in many cases where one eye has become deflected, as may appear from one to five years after birth. It is claimed that chiropractic has considerably minimized labor pains, save at ejection and after-birth . . ."

Chiropractors assert that even very young babies, in their process of getting acquainted with their environment by twisting and turning, are frequently prone to develop subluxations which in turn bring on many of the maladies of the formative years. For example, they say that even incontinence of bladder or bed-wetting may be corrected by spinal adjustment. Normally, chiropractors hold, a child develops proper bladder control at about two years of age. If this does not happen and bed-wetting persists without obvious cause, the trouble may not lie in the kidneys at all but in the bladder, where the sphincter muscle guarding the opening to the urinary canal is under control of the nervous system. In such cases a spinal subluxation is almost always present, and with adjustment the unusually prolonged incontinence vanishes.

Strenuous play, sitting for hours daily at desks, even carrying books to and from school in a habitual manner, as under one arm, is likely to cause postural faults and bring on subluxations in children, chiropractors assert. Records of absence from school show that children in the primary grades who are taught good posture have less illness. Yet, according to the recent White House Conference on Child Health, ". . . it is reasonable to believe that seventy-five per cent of the youth in the United States exhibits grades of body mechanics which are imperfect."

In recommending that every school child should be graded on his posture as much as on his deportment, arithmetic, or grammar, a well-known chiropractor, Dr. A. C. Johnson of Los Angeles, pointed out that "postural effects are no respecters of social or economic caste. Rich children, poor children, city children, and country kids all may suffer from postural defects.

"The posture of almost any given group of young people is uniformly bad. Yale and Harvard freshmen showed postural deformities in 85 per cent of the students. School children showed lateral postural defects in 34 per cent to 48 per cent . . . To get the best use of the human body, all its structures must be in proper alignment. Poor health may be found with no disease of an organ, but it is always associated with faulty alignments of the body."

The alarming prevalence of spinal deformity among our children was noted recently by Dr. Charles D. Napier of the House of St. Giles the Cripple, who conducted structural examinations of high-school girls in Brooklyn, New York. The *New York Times* reported that Dr. Napier found a high percentage of minor spinal, leg, and foot deformities. It quoted him as saying that spinal defects are more numerous among girls than among boys, and that early detection and care of the conditions might prevent serious trouble later. He emphasized that children of ten and twelve especially should be examined, for by the time they reach high school, it is sometimes too late to correct the condition.

Very recently, a group of research experts from New York University made structural checks of 6,400 typical children in twelve communities and found that 56 per cent of the group—representing both suburban and industrial areas—suffered from poor posture. It was predicted that backache, already rampant in the United States, would soon be even more prevalent than it is.

"Human spines were not evolved to withstand the monotonous, trying postures entailed by modern education," the great British anthropologist Sir Arthur Keith has observed. Along the same lines a well-known chiropractor noted acidly, "We have the turbine and jet-powered planes, the automatic windows in the new cars, gearshifts without clutches, color television, pop-up toasters. We are changing our environment more and more so that we will do less and less. Soon we may degenerate into a completely push-button existence. But our bodies are showing the results: most of us are beginning to look like slightly underdone muffins."

The plea that youths under the age of 19 should refrain from rugged, competitive sports because of the danger of possible injury to their still-developing spines was made not long ago at a meeting of the American Association for Surgery by the noted Chicago surgeon, Dr. John D. Ellis, who warned that:

"Change in shape of the bodies of the vertebrae occurs in young people from overexercise and competitive sports. This is particularly true in such sports as diving, football, and sometimes baseball, which cause powerful flexion and extension of the spine, and these diseases lead to a deformity of the back called 'adolescent angulation' or 'apprentice angulation.'

"Irreparable damage can be done by violent exercise involving powerful twisting of the spine in adolescence before the vertebrae are completely formed."

Much more along the same lines might be said, but this should be sufficient to show that not only the chiropractors, but many medical doctors as well, are aware of the importance of good posture in the prevention of disease and the part played by faulty posture in causing it. The case histories cited would seem to indicate that in the handling of a wide variety of children's ailments chiropractic is proving of great benefit, often after orthodox treatment has failed.

CHAPTER FOURTEEN

Chiropractic in Mental Ailments

There is a considerable accumulation of evidence that chiropractic is effective in the handling of various mental ills, perhaps even more effective in certain instances than the medical battery of treatment which includes psychoanalysis, psychiatry, drugs, various types of shock therapy, and surgery. This evidence has been piling up since the days of D. D. Palmer himself, who wrote that in the case of insane patients it was usual to find "occlusion of the third, sixth, seventh, eleventh, and twelfth dorsal nerves."

In 1952, a crusading book entitled *Obsolete American Mental Health Systems* made startling claims that both chiropractic and osteopathy were far superior to so-called "orthodox" procedures in the handling of mental ills. Written by John Stevenson, who was for many years a prominent figure in labor management in the State of Michigan, it made such direct comparisons as these:

"Under our present state mental health programs, seventy-five to ninety-five patients of every one hundred patients who enter state mental hospitals are doomed to an asylum prison for life, depending on which state the patients are confined in. The patient may be located in a state hospital where the average mental cure is the lowest per annum, beginning with Michigan, which has about one per cent cures per annum. Ranging across the nation to Massachusetts, we find approximately twenty-five per cent cures or satisfactory discharges. This costs the taxpayers $16,000,000 per annum in Michigan alone. Across the nation, involving every state, the total runs into hundreds of millions of dollars of the taxpayers' money . . .

"Investigation reveals that the private sanitariums of the chiropractic profession show from 60 to 65 per cent satisfactory discharges per annum as against 1 per cent to approximately 25 per cent discharges from state mental hospitals." (Italics author's.)

Stevenson charged that organized medicine maintains what amounts to a virtual monopoly over most state mental systems and mental hospitals, and stated: "There are very few hospitals employing chiropractors and osteopaths and they only in limited numbers. The legislators and governors of almost every state have failed to legislate osteopathic and chiropractic doctors for state mental hospital staffs. *The medical doctors and their associated psychiatrists would probably walk out of our state mental hospitals if our state legislatures enacted laws allowing chiropractic or osteopathic doctors to practice in state mental hospitals. The medicos would probably strike, the same as labor does when there's an unsettled issue with management."* (Italics author's.)

Stevenson also called for what he termed a "Tripartite State Mental Health System" in which each state should have at least one mental hospital operated

136

exclusively by chiropractors and one operated exclusively by osteopaths, in addition to the medically-operated setup. He has not progressed far in his campaign to date.

Over the years the increase in mental ills, ranging from those that do not incapacitate to those that require total care and in many instances restraint, has been steady and frightening. In 40 years prior to 1931, the total of inmates in U. S. state mental institutions climbed 460 per cent as compared with a population increase of only 110 per cent. In 1926, we had approximately 500,000 mental cases; by 1946, the total had reached almost 10,000,000, a twenty-fold increase in two decades. Both alcoholism and drug addiction—indications of emotional disturbance in the opinion of many authorities—have increased alarmingly.

In World War II, the chief reason for draft rejections and medical discharges by our armed forces was not, as might be supposed, some major killer such as heart trouble or cancer. Instead, it was mental illness. According to the U. S. Public Health Service, there are between 20 million and 30 million persons in this country who are "borderline" mental cases on the verge of "nervous breakdown."

Orthodox healers have consistently held the position that no connection exists between nervous breakdown and the nervous system. Their claim has been that there was no detectable difference between the nerves of the mentally calm and the mentally distraught. This position seems to be contradicted by the fact that chiropractic has had much success with "nervous breakdown" patients, who are so numerous and present a multitude of symptoms, such as irritability, insomnia, emotional flare-ups, muscular twitches, digestive disturbances popularly referred to as "nervous stomach," headaches, and a general apprehension about "cracking up."

Chiropractors state that clinical experience with many thousands of nervous patients has definitely established a direct connection between the nervous system and these disorders, demonstrating that the latter are not always of purely emotional origin. They also state that the physical alterations they are able to stimulate in the nervous system through spinal adjustment are highly successful in eliminating nervous symptoms, including those of long duration. This was stressed in a recent series of articles in the *National Chiropractic Association Journal* titled "The Connection Between Nerves and Nervousness" and written by Dr. Herman S. Schwartz, President of the National Chiropractic Psychotherapy Council and author of the popular self-help book *The Art of Relaxation.*

Now it appears that there is definite laboratory evidence of chemical differences between the nerves of persons who are tired and irritable and those who are rested and calm. The Swedish nuclear physicist Dr. Torbjoern O. Caspersson recently perfected a fantastically precise device which can detect changes in the protein content of individual human cells amounting to no more than one ten-thousandth of a gram in a cell of one-millionth of a meter in diameter. He has described as "profound" the chemical differences between the cells of persons who are tired and the cells of those who are rested.

Since tension and exhaustion almost invariably accompany "nervous breakdown" symptoms, the importance of the above discovery is obvious. According to Dr. Schwartz, Dr. Caspersson's findings "put to an absolute end the old argument—that since there are no *visible* nerve changes inside neurotics, the malady is strictly 'mental.' "

If chiropractic can do anything for patients with emotional and nervous disorders, then its record is worthy of attention. For, according to the Federal Security Agency's pamphlet *The National Mental Health Act and Your Community,* ". . . from 30 to 60 per cent of all patients consulting all doctors do so primarily for complaints due to emotional disorders . . ." And the U. S. Public Health Service, in a June, 1948, statement, admitted frankly that, "Our knowledge (of mental illness) is limited and many of our conclusions rest on slender foundations. We must learn more about the causes, treatment, and prevention of mental illness if we hope to improve the mental health of the people."

A valuable guide to the subject is a public-information booklet written by Dr. Schwartz with the technical and editorial collaboration of George W. Hartmann, Professor of Psychology, Teachers College, Columbia University. It is entitled *350 Nervous and Mental Cases Under Chiropractic Care* and was published by The Chiropractic Research Foundation of Webster City, Iowa.

Dr. Schwartz cogently sums up chiropractic's approach to mental illness. He says: "It is logical to ask how chiropractors correct nervous and mental conditions without resorting to psychiatry. The answer is that chiropractic is a neurological approach to these problems, operating on the independent assumption—

now an established scientific fact—that much emotional illness stems from nerve irritations maintained by distortions in the spinal column. By correcting these subluxations, the chiropractor eliminates intense and persistent pains of obscure origin which mental cases suffer. A person with a cinder in his eye sometimes shows temporary lack of emotional control. So does one who has his corn stepped on heavily. Perpetuate excitation with a less obvious source of trouble and one begins to understand why some of the mentally ill suffer."

Of the 350 patients in the Schwartz survey, 212 or 60.5 per cent were "apparently cured" through chiropractic, 87 or 25 per cent "much improved," 28 or 8 per cent "somewhat improved," 19 or 5.5 per cent revealed "no change," and 4 or 1 per cent were "worse."

Thus in 93.5 per cent of these patients improvement was noted ranging from apparent cure to some betterment of the condition.

"The summation here," observed Dr. Schwartz, "is that the chances are about 9 in 10 that 'nervous' cases of the sort considered, benefit from whatever the chiropractor does for them. Interestingly enough, *every one of the 350 cases studied revealed subluxations of variable magnitude in spinal analysis.*" (Italics author's.)

The Schwartz study becomes even more impressive when it is noted that of the patients studied 33 per cent had been in mental institutions and another four per cent were on the verge of being committed at the time chiropractic was first applied to them. More than 55 per cent had received general medical care, 13 per cent had undergone some form of shock therapy, and six per cent had had psychiatric treatment. Of the entire 350, all but five had had at least some degree of medical and psychiatric attention. Under such treatment, 27 or 8 per cent of the entire group had worsened, 33 or 10 per cent had shown some improvement, and 285 or 81 per cent had shown no change either for better or for worse.

Following are several cases from the Schwartz study:

General nervousness: G. I., age 26, married. Subject was employed as an assistant hotel manager. Duration of illness: 15 months. Subject complained of sick headaches, pains in his neck and behind his ears. He was extremely nervous and given to violent outbursts of temper without provocation. Inability to get along with people spelled a grave defect in his work and lessened job security. Subject's illness stemmed from a personal fight overseas in which he was knocked down. The medical officer who examined him at point of discharge from service heard the specific complaints. Eye glasses were recommended but brought no relief. Subsequently, under chiropractic care, the subject received 10 adjustments and was discharged in 1947 as apparently recovered. He re-enlisted in the Army and at last report was handling administrative duties capably without a sign of previous distress.

Neurasthenia: Male student, age 23. Illness was of 18 months' duration. Subject complained of severe head and back pains and imagined that he was suffering with a brain tumor. His mental condition was believed to have been precipitated by trying war experiences. Subject served in counterespionage for several years. This duty was of a consistently dangerous nature and held him in a state of high nervous tension over prolonged periods. Following the war, subject spent two months in a veterans facility and showed only partial improvement in this time. A throat specialist referred the case to a chiropractor in February, 1949. Subject responded favorably to the first of a series of adjustments and within six weeks was discharged as apparently recovered.

Schizophrenia: Male student, age 22. Violent and under guard. Suffered acute hallucinations. Accused family of trying to throw him into a lion's den. Under care of a number of M.D.'s who diagnosed case as acute mania. Papers signed for subject's commitment. Mother refused to have him committed. Patient came under chiropractic care in highly excitable state. M.D. administered anesthetic to facilitate vertebral analysis. Immediate improvement noted following first adjustment. Subject recovered in four weeks. Returned to college to complete studies.

Noting that "A community hospital belongs to all the people," Dr. Schwartz called for the inclusion of chiropractors on the staffs of such institutions. "In many forward-looking institutions," he wrote, "a therapeutic 'team' consists of a psychiatrist, psychologist, general medical practitioner, psychiatric nurse, social worker, and clergyman, all combined on the principle that the diversity of patient problems requires an organization of specialized skills. Add a chiropractor to the lineup, and the 'team' would be complete . . ."

One of the best-known chiropractic institutions dealing with the mentally ill is Forest Park Chiropractic Sanitarium in Davenport, Iowa. Its record in mental cases appears far superior than that of many, if not all, orthodox institutions. As far back as 1934, through the efforts of Hon. A. W. Ponath, County Judge of the Probate Court of Richland County, Wahpeton, North Dakota, 10 patients from the State Hospital at Jamestown, North Dakota, who had all been diagnosed as hopeless and incurable cases of dementia praecox, were sent to Forest Park in a test of what chiropractic could or could not accomplish. All of the 10 were chronic cases, and eight of the ten had been in the North Dakota state mental institution for from five to ten years. The remaining two were acute cases who had been mentally deranged for only a short time.

With these ten mental patients—all of whom had been diagnosed by state-employed medical doctors and psychiatrists as hopelessly incurable—Forest Park appears to have achieved 80 per cent complete recovery. The two acute cases were completely recovered by the end of the second month of treatment. Of the eight chronic cases, six were returned home as free from symptoms within one year.

Judge Ponath subsequently published a report titled *Facts—What Chiropractic Has Done for Insanity* in which he compared the overall records at Jamestown, N. D., (under medical supervision) and Forest Park (chiropractic). He found that during the years 1922-1934 the state mental hospital achieved 27.18 cures or satisfactory discharges, as compared with 65 per cent of the chiropractic institution over the same period.

Judge Ponath concluded, "And if this record, 65 per cent, can be obtained on cases where the large percentage are classed as incurable and had already spent much time in insane asylums and other sanitariums, how much more chiropractic could do if given the opportunity to handle the patients immediately after being brought to an insane asylum, rather than months or years later when their constitution has been run down by deterioration or prolonged mental disability or both."

According to a recent survey by the National Chiropractic Association, of a total of 2,556 cases of mental illness reported to the Association, 1,702 were completely restored to normal through chiropractic, 431 were partially restored, and 423 obtained little or no benefit.

Part Three

YOUR HEALTH AND THE INEVITABLE
ADVANCE OF NEW IDEAS

CHAPTER FIFTEEN

Organized Medicine's Private War Against Chiropractic

Since its founding in 1895, chiropractic has been noteworthy for the steady improvement in its educational standards, in the skills of its practitioners, and in the rapidly increasing millions of satisfied chiropractic patients. Under the circumstances, it would seem logical to conclude that medical doctors might be happy to welcome this new healing art, take note of its special approach to health, and refer patients to chiropractors when the patient's condition warrants.

Such acceptance has generally not been the case, even though the average medical doctor is overworked and admits privately to himself that there are many areas of illness in which he can be of little or no help. Although the total of M.D.'s who recommend chiropractic is increasing, it is still tiny compared to the entire profession, while the majority of medical doctors, following the lead of their official organizations, have very little, if anything, to say in chiropractic's favor.

There are several reasons for this. The first, to put it bluntly, is fear of successful competition. To recall the cynical comment of Horace Gray, M.D., in *New Inter-*

national Clinics: "It is well known that the regular physician seldom speaks favorably in public of any outside the regular fold."

Another reason, in many instances, is sheer ignorance of chiropractic, which seems usually to be accompanied by an unwillingness to accept and investigate the possibility that there might be a successful method of healing not taught in medical schools. This attitude of "if I don't know it, then it can't be of much value" is not limited to medical doctors; it is a common human failing.

The truth is that few medical doctors know anything about chiropractic. Most M.D.'s have not studied it, and it is seldom mentioned except disparagingly in medical journals.

This medical ignorance of chiropractic was emphasized scathingly in a recent article in *Medical Economics,* which asked the M.D. such questions as these:

"Have you or your medical society conducted any conclusive research to determine whether there's any validity in chiropractic doctrine? If so, what are the specific details? If not, what makes you so positive that there's nothing to chiropractic? What recent chiropractic textbooks have you read? Do you read the scientific articles in chiropractic journals? No? Then, since you admit your ignorance of progress in chiropractic, why do you come here as an expert on the subject?"

As the great English philosopher, Herbert Spencer, once observed, "There is a principle which is a bar against all argument, and which cannot fail to keep a man in everlasting ignorance. This principle is condemnation without investigation."

Spinal adjustment in the treatment of disease was not only unknown to the medical profession until recently, but was pooh-poohed besides.

In 1934, when a bill to license chiropractic was about to be introduced in the New York State Legislature, a questionnaire was sent to 29 men who were either medical doctors or who had studied anatomy in medical schools. Its purpose was to get their views regarding chiropractic.

One of the respondents, Dr. Charles Macfie Campbell, Director of Boston Psychopathic Hospital and Professor of Psychiatry at Harvard University, made no bones about his ignorance of chiropractic, but went right on to condemn it anyway. He wrote "I have made no independent study of the writing of those who represent the procedure called chiropractic, but my impression is . . . that it is based upon inadequate and misleading anatomical and physiological statements . . ."

Only three of the 29 respondents said they thought some illnesses might be caused by subluxated vertebrae. Only nine stated that they had first hand knowledge of how subluxations could cause narrowings of the vertebral openings. Only eight granted that subluxations might be reduced by hand. Only two said there might be some scientific basis to chiropractic.

The New York chiropractic bill did not pass, and numerous others which have since been introduced in that state have also failed to pass, due, say chiropractors, to the efforts of the powerful New York State medical lobby, which is determined to prevent the enactment of chiropractic legislation in that state. It is of interest, however, that all the chiropractic principles outlined in the 1934 questionnaire have since been accepted by medical science although not, of course, under the name "chiropractic."

It is also significant at this particular point to note that medical science, or at least the conservative branch of it which in general has ruled the field with an iron hand, has a long record of opposition to new developments. Many a medical pioneer was ruthlessly pilloried and has gained recognition for his theories and work only after a bitter struggle.

Consider, for example, the great anatomist Vesalius, who was ridiculed mercilessly when he attempted to describe the human body as it is actually constructed. Also castigated was William Harvey, after he asserted that the blood circulates throughout the body. Dr. Bodington, when he suggested that tubercular patients be exposed to fresh air, was laughed down as a faddist. Semmelweiss, whose work with puerperal fever is now world acclaimed, was held up to scorn when he recommended that careful hygienic measures be employed at childbirth; his persecution was so brutal that he went insane. The Royal Society of Physicians of London rejected the discovery by Marshall Hall of the reflex function of the spinal cord and brain. More recently, the Australian nurse Sister Kenny was assailed for her new—and successful—approach to the handling of poliomyelitis.

Thus the attack on chiropractic is nothing new. Orthodoxy seems to have a congenital antipathy toward the new, while the intellectually hidebound seem to have a special talent for working their way into positions of authority.

To begin to grasp the scope of medicine's war

against chiropractic—and it *is* a war—it is necessary to understand something of the nature of so-called "organized medicine," as distinguished from the individual medical doctor. For many centuries, medicine has had its private organizations, just as numerous other arts and sciences like architecture and law have had. One of the purposes of these organizations has been to gain various advantages for members; another is to thwart possible competition.

In the United States, the major medical organization is the American Medical Association. Affiliated with the A.M.A. and working in close cooperation with it are state and county medical societies. The A.M.A. has been termed one of the most powerful monopolies in world history. In his book *The Medical Trust Unmasked,* John L. Spivak calls it "the most powerful trust ever organized . . ." In the book *These Cults,* Annie Riley Hale denounces the A.M.A. as "the most colossal, the most all-inclusive publicity machine ever known." Incidentally, in a famous recent action both the A.M.A. and the associated Medical Society of the District of Columbia were convicted in Federal Court on charges of preventing patients from utilizing the services of healers of their choice.

In the 1880's, U.S. organized medicine succeeded in having all the states enact "Medical Practice Acts" which in almost every instance defined the practice of medicine as including just about everything under the sun the M.D. chose to do. These acts also prohibited non-medical persons from engaging in any form of healing—since that would be practicing medicine—and set up penalties for violations. In effect, they outlawed all new types of healing that might come along, even though they bore not the slightest resemblance to the practice of medicine, and made it possible to prosecute and penalize under the charge of "practicing medicine without a license." It was only through the weight of cumulative favorable public opinion that legislative recognition of certain non-medical healing arts such as chiropractic was achieved. Even today, as previously noted, chiropractic still has no legislative sanction in four of our states although it is widely practiced in all of them.

Organized medicine, working as a pressure group, has succeeded in gaining control of practically all governmental health functions and services, staffing them with its own members. There is not a tax-aided or tax-supported hospital that is not under medical control. In many of these hospitals it is impossible for any sort of healer other than an M.D. to gain professional entry, even though his services are not only requested but demanded by the patient.

In some states, the medical organization has obtained the passage of legislation prohibiting other than medical doctors from using the title "doctor" even though non-medical practitioners such as chiropractors have earned doctors' degrees. In other states the chiropractor can refer to himself as a doctor only if he qualifies the statement by the additional words "of chiropractic." Thus, in these states, the medical doctor is merely "Dr. John Doe" while the doctor of chiropractic is "Richard Roe, Doctor of Chiropractic."

Because of preferential laws like these, the very title "doctor" has been largely appropriated by the medical group, and is generally associated in the public mind with medical doctors only. As a simple test of this, ask any person whether or not a chiropractor is a doctor, and he will probably say no, although the opposite is the truth.

The average layman will find it hard to believe this, but organized medicine has what amounts to a virtual monopoly over the flow of news to the public concerning the healing arts. In 1937, the A.M.A. held a "special conference" at which "representatives of organized medicine in America, medical columnists, and science reporters exchanged views on ways and means to keep the public informed of progress in medical science." Actually this was an attempt to persuade the writers to submit voluntarily to A.M.A. censorship. How well it succeeded may be gained from the fact that, even today, almost all science writers abide by a code which in essence says, "Science editors are incapable of judging the facts of phenomena involved in medical and scientific discovery. Therefore they only report discoveries approved by medical authorities of rank, like Fishbein (Morris Fishbein, M.D., former editor of the *Journal of the American Medical Association*), or those presented before a body of scientific peers."

The censorship works this way. Editors are human beings, subject to error like everyone else. They do not profess to be authorities on healing. So, when a story that might be controversial reaches an editor's desk, he generally picks up the telephone and contacts a medical censor for an opinion. If the verdict is "don't run it" the story is killed.

Does this appear incredible? Then try to get an item in favor of chiropractic, for example, in your local newspaper, on a wire service, or in a magazine. The chances are overwhelming that you will fail. Cynics assert that many editors fear that if they fail to follow the advice of a medical censor their publications will lose valuable drug advertising. Whether or not this is true, it is certain beyond doubt that the majority of editors consider the medical censor the ultimate authority on what and what not to print concerning healing.

Thus, in addition to belittling chiropractic at every opportunity, organized medicine is able to exercise an almost complete blackout on the subject of chiropractic's possible merits in virtually every medium of public information.

Another powerful weapon against chiropractic is the instigation of prosecution for "practicing medicine without a license." As early as 1903, D. D. Palmer was arrested, convicted, and jailed for six months on this charge. Thousands of similar prosecutions have been brought against chiropractors over the years since then. In most instances paid agents are used. These persons deliberately try to entice chiropractors to perform medical services, such as prescribing drugs. Chiropractic patients have been subpoenaed in droves.

As chiropractic gained more and more satisfied patients who knew from personal experience that chiropractors do not practice medicine, the medical campaign of prosecution frequently boomeranged.

What happened in the State of California is a case in point. In just one year, 450 of approximately 600 chiropractors were hauled into court and convicted of practicing medicine without a license. They were given jail sentences or the alternative of a fine. Instead of choosing the fines, they chose to go to jail. This attracted so much public sympathy for the chiropractors that in 1922, when a bill to license chiropractors was put before the voters in a referendum, it was passed by a majority of 145,000, although in the election prior to the mass convictions a similar bill had been defeated by 1,500 votes.

In many of these California cases the sympathy of practically all concerned (with the exception of the complainants who were almost invariably medical organizations and not individual medical doctors) was obviously on the side of the prosecuted chiropractors. This sympathy was expressed in various ways creating situations that ranged from the humorous to explosions of blistering anger.

In Bakersfield, following the arrest and arraignment of a trio of chiropractors, Judge Bunnel observed that very few witnesses for the prosecution showed up. When he asked the sheriff the reason for this phenomenon, the sheriff explained: "Your Honor, the sheriff's office has been unable to catch the witnesses. They hide under beds and run out the back doors. They won't testify against these chiropractors." The case, like a multitude of others, was dismissed because of lack of evidence.

In Taft, following the arrest of five chiropractors, the prosecution requested that each man be placed under $1,000 bond. But the judge, who apparently approved of the right to use chiropractic, drawled: "I'm very sorry, but a goat got in last night and ate up all the bonds for $1,000, so we'll make it $100."

When five chiropractors were arrested in a single day at Long Beach, the indignant citizenry staged a giant protest meeting that was attended by more than 1,200 persons. One of the principal speakers at this meeting was a fearless M.D., Dr. E. C. Fortin of Los Angeles.

Protests against the high-handed prosecution of chiropractors flooded the newspapers. Many not only defended the chiropractors but also attacked the tactics of organized medicine with enthusiasm. A letter written by a Sacramento minister and printed in *The California Telegram* blasted angrily, "To our knowledge not one accusation, as a matter of record in California, has been brought against any chiropractor by any patient. Charges and convictions were based upon decoy evidence.

"The Medical Practice Law is the only law, we believe, on the California Statute books that requires hired, coached, trained spies to detect violators of the law . . . It is a crime to incite to crime. If chiropractic is criminal, is it not a crime to incite the practice of chiropractic?"

What went on in California was not unusual; it was paralleled in practically every state prior to the enactment of chiropractic legislation. In states where chiropractic has not yet obtained official sanction it is still going on.

Largest of these is New York State, with 3,000 chiropractors and some 3,000,000 people who have been under their care. Many New York chiropractors have been arrested; on one occasion there was a mass arrest of twenty-two. Of the 22, only four were brought to trial and were promptly acquitted, while charges against the remaining 18 were dismissed because of lack of evidence.

Sometimes the charges brought against chiropractors have bordered on the bizarre. In a recent New York case a woman chiropractor was indicted by a Grand Jury on charges that she had violated the Medical Practice Act merely by proclaiming herself to be a chiropractor in conversation, and on her business cards, and in the classified telephone directory. She was convicted. But ultimately a higher court held that use of the legend "chiropractor" does not imply that the user is a practitioner of medicine, that conceivably a chiropractor can render a treatment to the human body which is not the practice of medicine, and that maintaining an office for the practice of chiropractic was not in violation of the Education Law, under which the Medical Practice Act is administered.

In Louisiana, where chiropractic still does not have official sanction, a similar situation prevails. About half the state's chiropractors have been hauled into court on charges of "practicing medicine without a license." And in Massachusetts, in a typical recent case, two Greenfield chiropractors were found guilty on the same old convenient charge.

Every time the supporters of chiropractic press for the enactment of chiropractic legislation or for other recognition of chiropractic, as by insurance companies, the opposition of organized medicine is immediate and powerful. For example, when a bill to include chiropractors in the Federal Employees' Compensation Act was introduced during World War II, letters were received from many medical leaders blasting chiropractic in no uncertain terms. It was described variously as ". . . not only over the hill but I believe on the down grade . . ." "As far as I know, chiropractic has made no valuable contribution to science, art, literature, or anything else . . ." "The public should be protected against such ignorance . . ." "The passage of such a proposal would be a travesty on the high quality of medical service . . ."

And at the hearings, medical blockbusters such as these were exploded:

"Chiropractic . . . has no fixed meaning." "Contrary to well-established and easily demonstrable facts . . ." "The chiropractic theory of disease is too ridiculous to withstand any kind of experimental proof." "An old form of faith cure under a new name . . ." "A total misrepresentation of both the structure and function of those parts it attempts to explain." *"Subluxations of the vertebrae do not occur and even if they did they would not cause disease of any internal organ."* (The last sentence is italicized to emphasize its importance; in Chapter 15 there will be found quotations from many medical doctors in direct contradiction to this statement.)

And along similar lines, in 1950, when hearings were underway in the Congress concerning a bill to authorize the appointment of doctors of chiropractic in the Department of Medicine and Surgery of the Veterans' Administration, the head of the Washington office of the A.M.A. wrote the legislators: "The theory (of chiropractic) is not new. It has been advanced for years and if it had scientific value, it is reasonable to believe that it would have been recognized and the system developed by some of our universities . . . (it is) a form of treatment which obviously is not the best."

In the four states where chiropractic has still not attained legislative recognition the battle against such legislation goes on year after year with machine-like persistence, even though public approbation of chiropractic is increasing steadily and the ultimate defeat of organized medicine appears certain. Obviously this last ditch struggle is fought with desperation and includes attempts to influence not only the legislators but the general public as well. According to chiropractors, just about every pressure tactic and dirty trick known to the most skilled and unscrupulous political machines is employed.

Consider New York State, where chiropractors are optimistic of winning, as an example. There, a recent article in a county medical journal ridiculed chiropractic as *chiro-quack-tic* and appealed to the M.D.s to "stand united as one man in vigorous opposition to the licensing of chiropractic."

A pamphlet, titled *What Price Your Life?*, was also given widespread public distribution. Again, according to chiropractors, this booklet is a scare-type smear of chiropractic and chiropractors, full of distortions of the truth and absolute falsehoods which are disproved by the spoken words and published writings of medical authorities themselves.

"Danger ahead" screams *What Price Your Life?* in warning the public against the pending bills to license "chiropractic and other cultists." Chiropractors are defined as "persons who have nibbled at the fringe of medical knowledge." D. D. Palmer is ridiculed as a young grocer "who also peddled fish" and practiced as a "magnetic healer."

Great emphasis is placed on instructional evils in the early days of chiropractic, while improvements in chiropractic education are belittled.

There is a strong implication that chiropractic is frequently dangerous. "Excerpts" are given from the records of the Chief Medical Examiner of the City of New York:

"A ten-year-old boy has appendicitis. A chiropractor treats him for 'stomachache.' The boy dies.

"A five-year-old girl has a chiropractic 'adjustment' for 'sore throat.' She, too, dies—from diphtheria.

"A prominent attorney is treated for headache. Autopsy after death reveals a small hemorrhage at the brain's base. But hemorrhage didn't kill the attorney. An 'adjustment' that was supposed to relieve the headache produced the man's death by causing a broken neck."

The implication is also plain that many similar cases might be found "in the records of medical examiners, courts and coroners throughout the country."

No graver charges than the above can be imagined. Regarding these three cases, the records show that the ten-year-old boy died around 1920, the five-year-old girl in 1922, and the "prominent attorney" in 1942. These same three cases have been publicized again and again by organized medicine, both in medical journals and in the public press.

Chiropractors ask somewhat sarcastically why, if they are responsible for so many deaths, only three alleged instances have been found in the records of the Chief Medical Examiner of the City of New York over a period of more than 20 years, while not one has been found since 1942. And they point out that for every such case occurring under chiropractic, a thousand headlines such as "Dies Following Operation" and "Stricken After Inoculation" might be quoted that cast grave implications concerning the merits of medical treatment. "Patient for patient and disease for disease," they emphasize, "the death rate under chiropractic is much lower than it is under medicine."

It is significant that in none of the above three cases were criminal charges brought against the chiropractor concerned, proof positive of no evidence of malpractice. Furthermore, chiropractors charge that the case of the "prominent attorney," as described in *What Price Your Life?*, is an out and out falsehood.

Here is the chiropractic version of that death. The "prominent attorney" came home. He may or may not have been intoxicated. He went into his bathroom, slipped, fell, and broke his neck. A chiropractor who happened to live next door, a Dr. Rosenstein, was summoned. He examined the injured man and summoned an ambulance; *he administered no chiropractic adjustment.* At the hospital, the man was pronounced D.O.A. (dead on arrival). Examination by medical doctors disclosed that his neck was broken. Only the newspapers and organized medicine "convicted" Dr. Rosenstein of implication in the attorney's death.

"Upon the physician depends life itself," continues *What Price Your Life?* and then comes the warning, "When we cheapen medical standards by licensing cults, quacks, and chiropractors, we step backward toward the days of witchcraft and wizards."

Chiropractors retort that since chiropractic is not medicine, medical standards cannot be cheapened by chiropractic licensure.

Then comes the flat statement that the chiropractor has contributed nothing to science. Chiropractors denounce this as an outright lie, provable as such by references in medical literature itself.

What Price Your Life? features a "warning" letter

by Edward T. Wentworth, M.D., *President,* Medical Society of New York, which carries all the authority of royalty. Here is this pronunciamento in its entirety:

"Any licensure of chiropractors just because they have been practicing chiropractic, means elevation to professional level of those who have not met the qualifications. It means giving professional status, prestige and official stamp of approval to those who do not have the qualifications. It means a compromise between scientific thought and completely unscientific thought. There is no such thing as compromise between science and fraud. Science is based upon demonstrable relations of fact to fact, not once or occasionally by chance, but always. Fraud is circumvention of factual relations by deceit and trickery. One single admission of fraud into science, destroys science."

This letter does not equivocate; it denounces chiropractic as "completely unscientific" and "fraud." The chiropractic reply is that it constitutes out and out libel. And jubilantly chiropractors assert that, despite organized medicine's most vindictive efforts in New York State, they are winning their battle there as well as everywhere else.

The private war of organized medicine against chiropractic never ceases, whether or not the latter has attained legislative sanction. One of the favorite medical devices is ridicule, which is nowhere better utilized than in the book *Fads and Quackery in Healing* by Morris Fishbein, M.D. Fishbein unfairly describes the typical chiropractor as using language like "Chuesday" and "Thoisday" for Tuesday and Thursday and jerking the patient's head "until his head cracks" or pulling his leg, "depending on the particular school of chiropractic in which he was instructed."

In at least one instance, medical pressure has succeeded in "killing" a presentation favorable to chiropractic even after publication. This occurred after the book, *Finding our Place in Life,* a vocational guidance aid for children, came out. When the medical censors read it, they found that it contained a section on the merits of chiropractic and the career opportunities it offered. They protested to the Heckscher Foundation for Children, which had produced the book, and the chiropractic material was deleted from subsequent editions.

It might seem from all of this—and much more that might be added—that chiropractic is just about finished, so thoroughly discredited that the only chiropractic patients remaining are gullible ignoramuses or crackpots. But such is not the case, despite the most determined and persistent efforts of organized medicine to destroy this competitor science. To the contrary, chiropractic is healthier than ever before, it has more practitioners and patients, its prestige is greater, and it is firmly established as the world's second largest healing art.

Abraham Lincoln once said: "You may fool all of the people some of the time, and some of the people all of the time, but you can't fool all of the people all of the time." This appears to have occurred in the case of organized medicine's war against chiropractic. A vast segment of the public has been guided by results rather than by propaganda, and chiropractic's amazing growth has been the result of their satisfaction. Except in a few remaining isolated areas and instances, organized medicine's war upon chiropractic has signally failed.

CHAPTER SIXTEEN

Medicine's "Glass House"

For well over half a century, organized medicine has waged an unceasing campaign to put across the idea that the medical doctor is infallible. By means of a steady stream of newspaper and magazine articles, books and motion pictures, radio and television presentations, the legend of the omnipotent "Man in White" has been firmly implanted in the public mind. And by similar tactics, non-medical methods of healing have been cleverly belittled and ridiculed.

On the whole, this campaign has succeeded very well. When a patient dies, the relatives generally accept the medical doctor's regretful "I have done everything possible" without question. And when a medical doctor makes a mistake it is very difficult to prove it; the evidence is buried and few medical doctors are willing to speak of the errors of their colleagues.

A large segment of the public senses that the medical doctor is not half so infallible as he would have his patients believe, and dissatisfaction with medical results is frequently so great that criticisms of medical practice find their way into media of public information.

For example, one national magazine published an article describing the disillusioning experience of a man whose symptoms were diagnosed by ten different medical doctors as having been caused by ten different diseases. Only one of the ten M.D.'s, of course, could have been right but there is the possibility that all ten were wrong.

All through the history of medicine some of the most distinguished practitioners have been frank to admit the shortcomings of their profession. Hippocrates, the "Father of Healing," debunked the idea that medical doctors could work miracles by proclaiming, "If anyone believes medical art capable of performing more than nature allows, he is either mad or ignorant." This is in close accord with the chiropractic thesis that the chiropractor can merely adjust, while only nature cures.

Similarly, Dr. Oliver Wendell Holmes remarked somewhat sardonically that "Nature cures, but the doctor pockets the fee." He had scant respect for the efficacy of drugs and considered many of them more harmful than beneficial, saying: "If the whole *materia medica,* as now used, could be sunk to the bottom of the sea, it would be all the better for mankind—and all the worse for the fishes."

A great many medical men are opposed to the medical dependence upon drugs which has grown so prevalent in recent decades. The great medical pioneer, Sir William Osler, warned: "We put drugs, of which we know little, into bodies of which we know less, to cure disease of which we know nothing at all."

Dr. Harvey D. Cushing stated flatly that "a great part of what is called scientific medicine is a fetish."

166

Dr. James K. Hall observed, "Medicine has just about conquered all diseases only when we are talking to non-medical people," and added, "The most doleful and helpless mortal is the sick physician who has to subject himself to his fellow of like ignorance." And the famed anthropologist of Harvard University, Dr. Ernest A. Hooten, spoke of medical doctors as "high priests" who "patch up people but do not improve them."

"If we were honest, how many patients would we have?" asked Dr. William Howard Hay in commenting on medical guesswork. "Quacks" was his label for medical doctors who pretend to know exactly what they are doing when in fact they are in total ignorance of what to do.

In the light of observations like these, it is difficult to understand how medical propaganda such as *What Price Your Life?* can blandly dub chiropractic as "completely unscientific" and "fraud." There is an aphorism about the pot not calling the kettle black, and it seems to apply admirably to organized medicine's statements concerning chiropractic. Chiropractors do not denounce medical doctors as frauds, and they do not pretend to be infallible, even though, in many ailments, they achieve much higher percentages of cures than do the M.D.'s.

The chiropractor is not only concerned with diagnosing disease as a specific ailment. He searches for a detectable structural abnormality and corrects it. Thus wrong diagnosis to him is never a pitfall. The medical doctor, on the other hand, must make a correct diagnosis if he is to treat the patient effectively. When diagnosis is incorrect, medical treatment at best

167

does no good and at worst does much harm, if only in delaying application of the right treatment. As a result, any evidence of widespread error in medical diagnosis is highly disturbing, to say the least.

There is, unfortunately, a great deal of such evidence. One of the most important modern studies along these lines was made some years ago by Dr. Richard Cabot of Harvard Medical School. Dr. Cabot performed autopsies on the cadavers of patients who had died at Massachusetts General Hospital and found that more than 50 per cent of the diagnoses had been incorrect and that the patients had been treated for diseases they didn't have while there had been no treatment for the diseases they did have.

Dr. Cabot found 28 different fatal ailments in the cadavers he autopsied. In none of these ailments had diagnosis been 100 per cent accurate. It was highest for diabetes mellitus (95 per cent) and lowest for acute nephritis (16 per cent). In 13 of the ailments the percentage of correct diagnosis was 50 or less; these included chronic interstitial nephritis, thoracic aneurism, hepatic cirrhosis, acute endocarditis, peptic ulcer, suppurative nephritis, renal tuberculosis, bronchopneumonia, vertebral tuberculosis, chronic myocarditis, hepatic abscess, aortic pericarditis, and acute nephritis.

These findings emphasized what every medical doctor knows only too well, that correct diagnosis in some ailments is a simple matter while in others it is virtually impossible.

Many diseases are mistaken for others or are not detected at all. For instance, while serving as Surgeon General of the U.S. Public Health Service, Dr. Thomas

168

Parran made the startling statement that laboratory tests for syphilis were so inaccurate in this country that half of the cases of the disease were missed entirely while many persons who did not have syphilis were treated for it.

Incorrect diagnosis is undoubtedly responsible for millions of unnecessary surgical operations each year. "I am amazed at the discrepancy between the number of abdominal scars I see daily and the few cases of genuine acute appendicitis," Dr. M. G. Peterman told a recent meeting of the A.M.A. Dr. Norman F. Miller reported not long ago that 246 hysterectomies performed during a four-month period in 10 midwestern hospitals at least one-third had been unnecessary; he bluntly titled his report, which appeared in *American Journal of Obstetrics,* "Hysterectomy— Therapeutic Necessity or Surgical Racket?" Just as bluntly, the urologist Dr. Arbor D. Munger told an A.M.A. group that "In the surgical treatment of diseases of the kidney the fetish for nephrectomy (kidney excision or removal) comes near to being the surgical original sin." There are so many unnecessary operations on women that ethical M.D.'s refer to them as "rape of the pelvis." Operations performed solely for the purpose of making money and which are totally unnecessary are tagged "chronic remunerative."

Reporting in *Woman's Home Companion,* the well-known medical writer Albert Deutsch charged flatly: "Medical men have long known the shocking fact that nine million surgical operations performed annually in America are unnecessary. Among doctors it is an open secret that in many an operating room the cloak of surgery covers mayhem and even man-slaughter."

Sheer money hunger and not faulty diagnosis is responsible for innumerable unnecessary operations. According to Dr. Paul R. Hawley, director of the American College of Surgeons, this results in over-charging by numerous surgeons, fee splitting between surgeons and general practitioners, and even "ghost surgery"— a practice in which the patient believes that a prominent surgeon operated on him while actually the operation was performed by an assistant working for the big name.

It is possible for any hospital, by examining tissue after it has been removed, to determine whether an operation was necessary. Again according to Dr. Hawley, in some hospitals up to 70 per cent of the tissue removed in appendectomies was perfectly healthy. And in the report *American Medicine: Expert Testimony out of Court* appears the opinion that at least 50 per cent of the surgery performed in this country is the work of physicians who lack the "special qualifications" essential to first rate service.

The whole field of drug therapy is in a state of chaos, for many M.D.'s are completely bewildered concerning the merits or demerits of a wide variety of drugs. "Most drugs," wrote Sir William Osler, "have no curative effects whatever on the diseases for which they are administered." The famous *Baruch Report*— a study of so called "unorthodox" methods of healing financed by the wealthy statesman-philanthropist— stated unequivocally: "Medicine based exclusively on empirical use of pills and potions is becoming obsolete . . ."

There is a mountain of medical evidence that many drugs—in particular the new "wonder drugs" that are often rushed into widespread usage before their possible hazards are thoroughly investigated—have done a great deal of harm.

The world-famous pathologist, William Boyd, M.D., in his introduction of the recent 7th Edition (1961) of "A Textbook of Pathology, an Introduction to Medicine" makes a most revealing statement on this problem:

"Use of the library makes us aware of the fact that the picture of disease is changing before our very eyes. Old diseases are passing away as the result of the assaults of modern therapy, but new ones are continually taking their place. The inn that shelters for the night is not the journey's end. Many of these new diseases are iatrogenic (*iatros,* a physician) in nature; that is to say, they are the result of the well-meant but injudicious use of therapeutic agents. In these days when tranquilizers take the place of baby-sitters, blood transfusions are given thoughtlessly, indiscriminately and often needlessly, exposure to diagnostic or therapeutic ionizing radiation has become so universal, antibiotics are regarded as the cure-all for the most minor infections, and steroid therapy is the refuge of the destitute, it is small wonder that the old maladies are replaced by new man-made ones, and that allergies to a multitude of antigens have become so commonplace that they are said to exceed pathogenic microorganisms in number. I must apologize for the too frequent use of the words 'what is powerful for good can be potent for evil,' but this is true of so many situations created

171

by medical therapy that I have been unable to resist the temptation. If we continually interfere with nature, we must pay the penalty. The idea is of profound importance to the medical student who is to become the future doctor with the safety and welfare of his patient at heart."

Further, Robert H. Moser, B.S., M.D., associate professor of internal medicine, Graduate School, Baylor University, Houston, Texas, has just published a volume titled "Diseases of Medical Progress," which provides a startling survey of diseases and syndromes unintentionally induced as a result of widely accepted medical therapeutic procedures.

The survey lists dozens of diseases and fatal side effects and other hazards as a result of indiscriminate prescription of dangerous drugs in the following categories: antibiotic induced diseases, hormone induced diseases, collagen and collagen-like diseases, pulmonary diseases, renal diseases, cardiac diseases, metabolic diseases, dermatologic diseases, hematologic diseases, neurologic diseases, hepatic diseases and a number of other iatrogenic (physician-induced) diseases.

The Foreword of this book is startling in its frankness:

"It is no secret that certain drugs, surgical procedures, and other forms of therapy can, even when properly employed, create unfavorable, often harassing, and sometimes fatal side effects. Unhappily, it is also true that drugs are frequently administered or other procedures performed, apparently without due regard for their disquieting and sometimes dangerous potentialities. One need but mention, for example, the wide-spread use of antibiotics for trivial upper respiratory infections and comparable minor ailments—a practice that seems to continue in spite of the exhortations of many qualified authorities that these agents are, as a rule, ineffective in such cases."

And along the same lines *The New England Journal of Medicine* warned in its January 12, 1950, issue that although folic acid brings about remission in pernicious anemia, paralysis may be induced; that benadryl, employed against anaphylactic symptoms, may cause urticaria; that aminopyrine has caused many deaths and that *the toxicity of this drug was not proven until it had been in medical usage for 15 years.*

Penicillin is a proven killer and has probably taken far more lives than the official records indicate. The sulfa drugs have killed many thousands. In the treatment of pneumonia, sulfa was found to have killed one of every 160 patients treated with it. A U. S. Public Health survey revealed that the use of sulfa in treating burns, wounds, and ulcers often resulted in symptoms of sulfa poisoning such as severe skin eruptions.

Another "miracle drug," streptomycin, has been found to be nowhere nearly so efficacious as it was first believed to be. In tuberculosis, for example, it fails to benefit the majority of patients and may cause permanent vertigo, while the mere fact of its use often induces in the patient a false sense of security which may prove disastrous.

Still another "miracle drug," chloromycetin, was recently found to induce aplastic anemia which is frequently fatal. ACTH or cortisone has produced extremely grave complications in arthritic patients; one study of 4,376 patients treated with ACTH revealed that 734 had to be taken off the drug because of harmful side effects ranging from water-logged tissues to perforated ulcers. Thirty-five of the patients died of causes the investigators believed "to be directly attributable to the side effects of ACTH."

Hormones have been supposed to be wonder workers, too. But, according to the prominent health columnist Dr. T. R. Van Dellen, the female sex hormones "are not curative (in disorders of the female glandular system)" and prolong the climacteric or change of life adjustment. In both sexes, hormone treatments may stimulate the growth of cancer cells.

There is a great deal of evidence that "shots" and vaccines are nowhere near so effective as their boosters claim. One medical school of thought holds that the decline of many once prevalent diseases is actually due to improvements in general health through better diet and modern sanitation.

We have had some very dismal experiences following mass inoculations, particularly in the armed services, which indicate that the serums can sometimes cause more illness than they prevent. As a glaring illustration, during less than seven months of 1942, 28,585 cases of yellow jaundice broke out in U. S. soldiers following inoculations against yellow fever. It is a proven fact that smallpox vaccine has taken many lives. Following a 1947 "smallpox scare" in the New York area, six million persons were vaccinated. Shortly afterward, numerous deaths were reported from after-effects of the vaccine such as inflammation of the brain and spinal cord. In his May 14 broadcast, Walter Winchell declared that ". . . an unofficial survey indicated that more people died from vaccination than smallpox itself in the past months."

The subject of vaccines and inoculations is a medical hot potato. No less a medical power than the president of the Ohio Medical Society, Dr. J. F. Baldwin, came out with the assertion that "the hand that rocks the vaccine factory is the hand that rocks the medical profession." He was promptly deposed from his high post, which might indicate to some that what he said was absolutely accurate.

The drug industry is a billion dollar business, and unquestionably it wields tremendous power in the medical world. According to Dr. Charles Solomon in his paper *Chaos in Drug Therapy—A Vicious Circle,* big business competition and high pressure salesmanship by the drug manufacturers are responsible for a very sorry situation. "When . . . (the M.D.'s) credulity is played upon by subtle advertising psychology, and when the drug industry is so organized that ruthless profit competition occurs," he writes, "the results are disastrous not only to medical therapy but to pharmacy, to nursing, and to the teaching of pharmacology and related subjects."

There is no doubt that a vast number of medical doctors are either cynical about the alleged merits of a vast variety of drugs or follow the drug manufacturers' propaganda without question. They get on the bandwagon for every new "miracle drug" and prescribe it indiscriminately, knowing that their patients will consider them behind the times if they don't.

Furthermore, there is a growing tendency for M.D.'s to prescribe proprietary medicines (drug preparations with trade names) instead of working out prescriptions to fit individual cases. Because of the plentitude of proprietary medicines, it is a fact that many M.D.'s are extremely rusty in their *materia medica*. When your medical doctor writes a prescription "it is all too often written incorrectly," according to Dr. Solomon. This inaccuracy is a standing joke among druggists.

Also because of the tremendous variety of proprietary medicines that are available, many medical students neglect the study of *materia medica*. As internes, they are often "altogether incapable of writing a satisfactory prescription for a patient," an article in *International Medical Digest* charged some years ago. "The shelves of some hospital pharmacies remind one of the exhibits of proprietary medicines in a chain-drug-soda-fountain-lunch-room" wrote Dean Ernest E. Irons of Rush Medical College in *American Journal of Pharmacy*. Most trademarked drugs, according to Dr. Irons, cost far more than the standard drugs, although they do no more than meet the standards of the United States Pharmacopoeia. Thus a multitude of patients pays unnecessarily high prices for medications simply because their medical doctors are too ill educated, too lazy, or too busy to prepare individual prescriptions.

Nowhere is this professional flabbiness more evident than in the widespread prescribing of sedatives and narcotics which relieve pain and mask symptoms without effecting any benefit. According to Dr. Harry Gold, there is no depressant drug "in common use in which as a result of prolonged use there fails to arise a state of irritability and emotional unrest," while discontinuance of these drugs may result in symptoms ranging from irritability to convulsions.

Closely akin to the mumbo-jumbo of the witch doctor is the widespread administration of placebos or "little pink pills" which contain no drugs and whose sole benefit is psychological. Obviously the M.D. who passes out placebos along with some words of encouragement doesn't know what else to do. But, according to Dr. Wallace Y. Yater, chairman of the A.M.A. section on experimental medicine and therapeutics, placebos have no particular "psychological value" while the patient "should know what he is getting . . ."

Thus it is painfully apparent that incompetence and chaos exist in many areas of medical practice. The facts justify the statement of Waldemar Kaempffert, noted science writer of *The New York Times,* to the effect that medicine is "the most pretentious of all the sciences, and the least scientific . . ." They justify the cynical remarks that have been attributed to many medical doctors, such as the comment of a New York heart specialist that his work consisted mainly of "correcting the mistakes made by other doctors," or the remark of another prominent M.D. that the one action that would do most to improve medical services would be to "chloroform half the medical profession."

So the infallible "Man in White" does not appear to be so infallible after all. Under the circumstances, it is not surprising that medicine is losing patients to chiropractors by the millions. If the medical doctor spent more time in improving the quality of his own services and less time in belittling and even libeling a successful competitor, say chiropractors, everybody would be benefited.

As *Medical Economics* observed: "Do you (the M.D.) think the average American is too ignorant to know what's good for him? If not, why not let him decide whether he wants to go to a chiropractor? . . . Isn't that the American way?"

FROM HEALTH AND CHIROPRACTIC

CHAPTER SEVENTEEN

*Medical and Lay Opinions
in Favor of Chiropractic*

One of the great stores of the world is Bergdorf-
Goodman's, in New York City. Much of the success
of this store has been due to the immense energy and
continuing good health of its president, Edwin Goodman, over many years. When Mr. Goodman reached
his 75th birthday, naturally a first rate party was
held in his honor. Among those present was the well
known publisher Dorothy Schiff. Intrigued by Mr.
Goodman's exuberant health, she asked him for his
secret so that she might pass it along to younger
people.

"Just get yourself a good chiropractor," advised
Goodman.

That was brief and to the point. No equivocation,
no hedging. Millions of persons feel the same way
about chiropractic and are equally enthusiastic in its
praise. They come from all walks of life and all
stations in life. Some are of average education like
most of us, but many are of the highest intellectual
background, a fact which challenges the medical
propagandists' claim that chiropractic patients are
ignorant and gullible.

179

Scores of testimonials to chiropractic appear in Part Two in the form of quotations from enthusiastic patients, most of whom were cured by chiropractic after medical treatment had failed. They disprove the frequent medical assertion that "all that science can do is being done," and prove conclusively that "all that science can do is not being done unless chiropractic is provided." Most of the testimony cited in Part II came from the so-called "little people"—those who have made no great mark in the world and whose names are unknown outside their own communities and personal circles. But the same kind of enthusiastic praise of chiropractic comes also from men and women who stand above the crowd, ranging from governors to leaders of finance and industry and including not a few prominent medical doctors. Indeed, there is a great deal of pro-chiropractic testimony in the medical literature itself.

Regardless of his education and station in life, nobody knows better than the sick person himself that he is sick, when he starts to get well, and who is responsible for his improvement. On these points the testimony of the humblest common laborer has equal validity with the testimony of the world celebrity. However, to refute the charge of certain medical doctors that chiropractic patients are ignorant nonentities, we should examine the statements of persons distinguished in our society.

Elbert Hubbard, who wrote "A Message to Garcia," was a very famous American author, editor and publisher. Hubbard was one of the earliest chiropractic patients and became a crusader for this healing art. He wrote a book on good health measures, titled *The*

Science of Keeping Well, in which he declared:
"Chiropractic never brings an adverse result. The
chiropractor does not pin his faith in any single
panacea. He simply knows the physical fact that a
pressure of bone on the nerve brings about a condition
where the telegraph system fails to act properly. With
skilled hands he brings about the right relationship
and proper adjustment. He finds the cause and re-
moves it. Chiropractors are not doctors of medicine.
They are doctors of health. From them we get a new
science which is adding greatly to the happiness and
welfare of the world."

Many other writers have written favorably of chiropractic after personally experiencing its benefits.
Typical is the Minneapolis *Tribune* columnist, Cedric
Adams. He had come down with laryngitis and had
undergone a variety of medical treatment. Yet, after
three weeks, he was still a "whispering baritone."

At this point, a woman phoned him and told him
how Senator Burton K. Wheeler of Montana had been
cured of laryngitis by a St. Paul chiropractor. He decided to try chiropractic. "In exactly two treatments,"
he wrote in his column, "I am almost back to normal
voice, so today, heresy or no, I salute chiropractic with
this personal testimonial."

In the field of politics, U. S. Senator Glen Taylor
had a similar experience. He was introduced to chiropractic by his wife, who was already a chiropractic
patient, after he suffered a subluxation which made it
impossible for him to stand up. After a few chiropractic adjustments—he didn't recall the exact number but he did recall that there weren't many—he
wrote his chiropractor, "My back has never bothered

me since, and I have done many different kinds of work, including two years manual labor in an unheated war plant . . . I never miss an opportunity to tell my friends of the truly remarkable service chiropractic has rendered us."

Of the governors and other leading officials of the various states, the following are some who have written favorably of chiropractic:

ARKANSAS ". . . the law which has been passed in this State governing the practice of chiropractors is very satisfactory to the public in general, and which law places such practitioners upon a very high standing and much better than formerly." H. W. Appelgate, *Attorney General.*

ARIZONA ". . . (chiropractic) practitioners of high standard." John W. Murphy, *Attorney General.*

COLORADO "From what I know of the chiropractic profession in Colorado, I would say that its operations have been satisfactory." John C. Vivian, *Governor.*

CONNECTICUT ". . . there have been few complaints in regard to the operation of the chiropractic law in Connecticut." Stanley H. Osborn, *Commissioner, Department of Health.* (In Connecticut, the Health Commissioner is a medical doctor.)

DELAWARE ". . . many people believe in it and have assured me that they or some of their families have been benefited by this treatment." Richard C. McMullen, *Governor.*

GEORGIA ". . . the chiropractors have apparently become quite popular in Georgia." T. R. Gress, *Asst. Attorney-General.*

IDAHO (Letter to a chiropractor) "I wish to assure you of my appreciation for the work being carried on by the members of your profession." Barzilla W. Clark, *Governor*.

Iowa "The practice of chiropractic in this state is now a matter of pride, not only to those engaged in the practice, but also to the state as a state." Ben J. Gibson, *Attorney-General*.

Kentucky "Chiropractors are doing their work in every civilized country of the world and those who feel that they have been benefited through the science and philosophy of chiropractic are legion. Every healing agency should have the sympathetic interest and support of us all." Albert D. Chandler, *Governor*.

Missouri "We feel, here in Missouri, that the Chiropractors have a distinct work to do and they are doing it, and we consider the bill giving them a license as one of the forward steps in legislation." Sam A. Baker, *Governor*.

Nevada "The chiropractic profession has cooperated with the health authorities in the maintenance of sanitary and quarantine safeguards and in the control of epidemics. They have the same standing and fees paid to M.D.'s by the Industrial Commission." E. P. Carville, *Governor*.

New Hampshire "The great numbers of those who today practice the science and art of chiropractic may derive great satisfaction from a contemplation of the great progress that has been made . . . Chiropractic was introduced to the people of New Hampshire in 1915 by a single chiropractor in the City of Manchester . . . By this time chiropractic has spread to every city in the state and many of the smaller communities . . . Any art, science or service which is helpful to the suffering is a credit to itself and deserves public commendation. This I am glad to accord to chiropractic." Francis P. Murphy, *Governor.*

NEW JERSEY "We have many chiropractors in our state, and they must be rendering service to suffering humanity or they would not be able to continue." A. Harry Moore, *Governor.*

NEW MEXICO "Many of our most enlightened citizens avail themselves of the chiropractic form of healing . . ." R. C. Dillon, *Governor.*

NORTH DAKOTA ". . . I do not believe the practice of chiropractic is in any way embarrassing to practitioners of the regular medical profession." A. G. Sorlie, *Governor.*

OKLAHOMA "This state has a Chiropractic Board, and it is functioning splendidly." H. E. Sullivan, *Secretary to the Governor.*

OREGON "I have reason to believe that the Oregon Law regulating the practice of chiropractic has the approbation of the general public and practitioners of all branches of therapeutics." Walter M. Pierce, *Governor.*

SOUTH DAKOTA ". . . The South Dakota Chiropractic Law has been beneficial to the citizens of the state and has also elevated the class of individual practitioners." Benjamin J. Mintener, *Assistant Attorney-General.*

UTAH "The operation of the chiropractic law in the State of Utah is very satisfactory due to the high standards of requirements fixed by the State Board of Chiropractic Examiners . . ." Rena B. Loomis, *Assistant Director, Department of Business Regulation.*

WASHINGTON ". . . the people in general are well

pleased . . ." Charles R. Murphy, *Director, Department of Licenses.*

(Also available are many favorable comments from state boards of chiropractic examiners.)

Whenever chiropractic legislation has been proposed, both individual members of the laity and organized groups go on record as in its favor. As an example, when a bill to amend the Federal Employees' Compensation Act by the inclusion of chiropractors was introduced in the U. S. Congress, ten major organizations went on record as endorsing the bill. These were: American Federation of Government Employees, National Federation of Federal Employees, National Federation of Post Office Clerks, National Association of Letter Carriers, National Association of Railway Mail Clerks, Washington Branch Railway Mail Association, Baltimore Branch Railway Mail Association, Huntington (W. Va.) Railway Mail Association, The Community Councils of the City of New York, and Virginia State Federation of Labor. Several letters from medical doctors endorsing the bill were introduced into the record.

Legislators favoring chiropractic laws have frequently made powerful and highly logical pleas on chiropractic's behalf. Typical is the presentation delivered before the New York State Assembly on the last day of its 1942 session by Assemblyman Orlo M. Brees of Broome County:

"Merely to make it clear to this House once and for all the difference between the chiropractors and the medical fraternity, and I have the highest respect for the great majority of them, let me illustrate it from the field of mechanics. Gentlemen, if you are

185

driving your automobile and the front wheels are out of alignment, you may have the finest chemists in the world who can give you the octane rating of gasoline, but they cannot correct the misalignment by prescribing a change of fuel. That is a mechanical job requiring a mechanic. In the healing field the chiropractors are the mechanics, and the medical practitioners are the chemists, and there is plenty of room for both of them; but the administration of drugs will not correct a structural misalignment or distortion . . ."

This is one of the simplest yet clearest presentations of the difference between medicine and chiropractic ever made by anybody. The medical doctor is indeed the chemist and the chiropractor the mechanic, but in both instances superlative training and skill are taken for granted, for the human body is the most complex assemblage of chemical compounds and the most intricate array of interworking mechanisms that we know of.

In cases where chiropractors have been brought into court on charges of practicing medicine without a license (See Chapter Fifteen, *Organized Medicine's Private War against Chiropractic*), the court has gone out of its way to praise chiropractic. As far back as 1920, Judge Lansden of the Supreme Court of Tennessee said:

"The Court thinks that Chiropractors cannot be classed along with charlatans and fakirs. It is a well-developed system of healing, recognized in many jurisdictions, and many believe in its efficacy . . ."

Similarly in Illinois, the case of *People vs. Love, 298 Illinois, 304,* the Illinois Supreme Court observed:

"It is not the province of the courts to extol or

belittle chiropractic, osteopathy or medicine and surgery. They are all now established as useful professions, and as time has progressed it has been thoroughly demonstrated that all of them have accomplished, and all are daily accomplishing, the relief and cure of human ailments.

"Constantly comes proof before the courts that chiropractic does enable the chiropractor to relieve and cure many of the ailments of human beings, and that the practice of this science is in no way deleterious to the human body. That is the proof in this record." In this decision, incidentally, the Illinois Medical Act was declared unconstitutional.

Numerous medical doctors who have become chiropractors have added their praise, which is of great value since these M.D.'s have had the unusual experience of comparing the two healing arts with well-trained and scientific exactitude. For example, Dr. A. Walton, after studying chiropractic, wrote, "For the first time in the history of the world we have chiropractic, a system which is dignified and scientific in principle; therefore, if one must be conservative, do not be paleozoic and persist in clinging to obsolete methods."

Similarly, after studying chiropractic, Dr. M. E. King wrote in *Therapeutic Review*: "There was a time when I looked at chiropractic through a pair of bifocal lenses, the upper plus prejudice, the lower plus lack of investigation . . . I went . . . to a school of chiropractic and, to my surprise, they were actually getting results on cases that were hopelessly incurable from the standpoint of medicine. I soon saw that the theory that they were working on was plausible and had the approval of common sense. All this opened up a new field of thought to me which had never been presented through the study of medicine. The sooner the medical profession recognizes the work of the chiropractor, the better. He is doing a work that medicine cannot do; he belongs exclusively to the class of specialists and should be recognized."

The New York City orthopedist Dr. La Forest Potter declared, "After practicing medicine fifteen years and spinal adjustment nearly ten, I am daily astonished at the power of spinal adjustments as a cure for disease."

The British team of Osgood and Morrison referred frankly to "brilliant and rapid . . . chiropractic cures." Dr. R. F. Allendy admitted the chiropractic thesis that "considerable organic effects" result from subluxations. Dr. H. B. Gotten considered it better that the chiropractor treat low-back pain cases than "the physician who thinks only in terms of surgery." One reason for the popularity of chiropractors, in the opinion of Dr. H. T. Hyman, was the "failure of the medical profession to provide this type of service."

In his book *Eugenics,* Dr. H. H. Rubin declared that a considerable variety of symptoms "may be due to nothing more serious than a displaced vertebra, which any competent . . . chiropractor can restore to normal position in ten seconds . . ." Dr. Hartwell, a president of the New York Academy of Medicine, speaking in his official capacity before the Board of Regents of the State of New York, frankly admitted that chiropractic has a real value in the treatment of disease.

Dr. Adolph Lorenz, son of the world famous Viennese surgeon, described chiropractic as "a blessed substitute for the usual reparatory methods" in bone misplacements. "What is the matter? Why have we failed when the chiropractors have succeeded?" wrote Dr. B. V. Watts. Dr. J. A. Fischer admitted that ". . . the results obtained with spinal adjustment are phenomenal." In *Medical Economics* appeared this devastating (to the orthodox M.D.) paragraph: "In treating backache the general practitioner may do a pelvic examination, find a cervical erosion and perhaps send the patient to a surgeon for cauterization. When this fails to bring relief, the surgeon does an operation of hysterectomy. Eventually the patient goes to a chiropractor. In five minutes the chiropractor may find that the patient has a postural backache and in fifteen minutes may have succeeded in cutting the ground from under the G.P. and the surgeon. Thus a chiropractic convert is born."

Dr. J. Mennell admitted in his book *The Science and Art of Joint Manipulation* that ". . . so long as the medical profession withholds this method of treatment, so long will patients seek the advice of manipulators outside the profession . . ." And Dr. H. W. Scott, after writing that he examined the spines of all patients, admitted that he obtained his knowledge of vertebral abnormalities and their correction "from a chiropractic college."

Dr. B. Gomroe, of the University of Pennsylvania Medical School, declared concerning low-back symptoms in his book *Arthritis and Allied Conditions,* "They respond well to manipulative measures. It is this type of patient who may be 'miraculously cured' by certain mechanical maneuvers of Chiropractors which are frowned upon and looked askance at by the medical profession."

Finally, Dr. George S. Weger wrote that he was personally acquainted with many very excellent medical doctors who patronize chiropractors. This strikingly parallels the experience at "German Therapy Week" in 1953 when, as described in Chapter Two, Dr. Karl Sell was besieged by medical doctors who wanted chiropractic adjustments following a lecture on chiropractic.

A sound evaluation of chiropractic has been made in the Canton of Geneva, Switzerland, where chiropractic has been regulated for some time. Mr. Claude Ketterer of the House of Deputies recently made the following observations:

"Now the domain of static troubles of the vertebral column and of diseases of vertebral origin is specifically that of chiropractic. Chiropractors have studied these questions for several decades and their researches have been directed in this direction. Since the end of the last century, they have been taking care of these affections by specific manipulative treatments, and they were among the first to occupy themselves therewith. Dr. J. Terrier, medical specialist in rheumatology at Baden, Switzerland, has expressly recognized this. (*Bulletin des medecins suisses*, No. 9, 1959.)

"It would be truly incomprehensible and unjustifiable to continue to exclude chiropractors, who are the real specialists in this domain, from commissions concerned with public health. On the contrary, they will be able to bring thereto their competent contribution to a domain which does nothing but grow.

"For a number of years, the publications in the chiropractic domain of affections of vertebral origin have been multiplying at an extraordinary rate. To this alone, the collection of Professor Junghans, who is trying to gather together all the works and publications bearing on the domain of the vertebral column and its affections, had reached by 1960 the impressive figure of 203 titles. This domain is becoming more and more a *scientific specialty*. Neither the general medical practitioner nor the medical specialist of another medical domain today has the possibility of knowing well enough the special domain of chiropractic. It is a question of a specialty which has remained outside medicine, but of capital importance for public health, in which the only experts are the chiropractors."

It is obvious from all the above that the supporters of chiropractic are now legion indeed. The growing recognition of chiropractic in many walks of life—including the medical profession—and the praise freely accorded chiropractic by a highly diversified cross-section of the American public, undoubtedly explains in considerable degree why chiropractic is expanding at the rate of two million new patients a year. "Let a man build a better mousetrap, and the world will beat a path to his door, even though he live in the depths of the forest."

CHAPTER EIGHTEEN

Medicine's About-Face

At the time D. D. Palmer began adjusting the spines of the first chiropractic patients, organized medicine was quick to denounce spinal adjustment as unscientific and worthless, as well as dangerous. That attitude has persisted. Curiously enough, however, over the decades many medical practitioners have not only "discovered" the existence of spinal subluxations and their influence on health, but they have made definite attempts to develop forms of spinal manipulation of their own.

Many a fairminded M.D. must have asked himself the question, "Are we trying to steal chiropractic without giving credit where credit is due? If imitation is the sincerest form of flattery, aren't we demonstrating our belief in chiropractic's value more and more while still condemning what we imitate?"

An examination of medical literature reveals amazing medical ignorance, until recent years, of the spine and of the effects of spinal subluxations upon the nervous system and the body's resistance to disease. Early medical attempts to reduce subluxations were unbelievably crude by comparison with chiropractic techniques. This medical backwardness in the field of body mechanics has persisted to the present, chiropractors hold, and is due to the fact that the basis of medical practice is drug therapy.

Many medical authorities deny flatly that subluxations could occur, or, if they did occur, that they could be adjusted by hand. Mention has already been made of the responses by medical men to a New York State questionnaire specifically requesting their opinions of chiropractic; the overwhelming majority were opposed to both chiropractic theory and practice. Possibly their answers were colored by prejudice; but many such opinions must also be considered to have been the result of ignorance, and of failure to research the field scientifically.

Thus, Dr. Louis S. Reed asserted that vertebrae are dislocated only rarely and that pressure by them upon the spinal nerves is "practically impossible." Dr. Dean Lewis, Surgeon-in-Chief of Johns Hopkins Hospital, stated that, in his opinion, spinal subluxations could not be reduced by hand. Dr. R. Bensley, Director of the Department of Anatomy of the University of Chicago, stated that in a period of 29 years he had never observed a single instance in which spinal vertebrae had caused pressure upon nerves. Dr. J. B. Roberts wrote that sacroiliac subluxations "must be rare" since the medical textbooks contained few instances of them. Magnuson and Coulter noted the general medical belief that the sacroiliac joint was immovable.

But—and often almost simultaneously—directly opposed viewpoints have been appearing with increasing frequency in medical literature. As far back as

1911, Dr. R. O. Meisenbach stated that sacroiliac "joint strain" was more common "than generally supposed." In 1913, Dr. R. Fitch described a case of lumbo-sacral subluxation "accompanied by nerve pressure." In 1914—in a *Medical Record* paper that attracted widespread attention and provoked a great deal of controversy—Dr. J. H. Radley wrote: "The possibility that not a single medical man has ever palpated a spinal subluxation or witnessed its correction and the results thereof is no proof at all that such a condition does not exist. One convincing, positive demonstration outweighs in evidential value all the speculation, yes, scientific negation that can be accumulated. In literature reaching the hands of the recognized medical profession, there is such a scarcity, as to amount to almost a complete absence, of matter dealing with spinal subluxations; and of that which comes to their notice, practically all of it is so misinforming and misleading as fully to account for the almost universal denial, by physicians, of the possible existence of such a condition . . . That spinal subluxations are of frequent occurrence; that they attend, if they do not precede and cause, disease in remote tissue; and that correction of these lesions is followed by restoration to normal condition and function of such remote tissue (at least subjectively to the patient, as evidenced by the disappearance of symptoms), are all matters of repeatedly demonstrated fact."

Generally, however, orthodoxy, inertia, and a reluctance to investigate revolutionary new ideas continue to dominate medical thinking on the subject of subluxations. Dr. E. J. Carey noted that "too frequently" medical students neglected the anatomy of the back. Sardonically, Dr. T. A. Willis observed that in the course of dissections, very few students showed curiosity regarding spines while the average surgeon had a propensity for turning his female patients over and removing "some of the dispensable parts from the abdomen or female pelvis, concerning the anatomy of which his curiosity has naturally been more active." The average surgeon "does not understand" back cases, wrote Dr. J. E. Goldthwait. Dr. G. Mitchell warned of "widespread ignorance of the anatomy of the lower back and the mechanics of the lower spine." In no field of medicine was there "greater ignorance" than concerning backache, stated Dr. R. H. Paramore.

By the mid-1920's, medical references to subluxations and their effects on spinal nerves and in disease were quite frequent. In 1935, Stimson and Swenson referred to "sudden and spectacular increase" in medical reports of subluxations. The following year, Pitkins and Pheasant reported finding sacroiliac subluxations in 326 (64 per cent) of 506 patients. Now the medical doctors were really commencing to look for subluxations—and finding plenty of them.

Belatedly, the medical viewpoint was coming around to resemble that promulgated by Palmer. A variety of ills as well as "multiple vague symptoms" were simply "phenomena of crooked spines," wrote Atsatt and Atsatt. "Many disabilities, formerly classified as lumbago back strains, etc., are now being recognized as due to displacements," stated Dr. H. J. Ullmannin in 1924. A decade later, Dr. A. B. Ferguson wrote that spinal displacements were "commonly associated with symptoms." Over the years, various M.D.'s wrote of arthritis, rheumatism, neuralgias, adbominal pains,

195

lumbago, headaches, nervous irritability, low-back pains, and a multitude of other ills being associated with subluxations.

Within the medical camp there was also growing recognition not only that subluxations can and do exist but that they also cause pressure on nerves, and that this pressure causes interference in the flow of nervous impulses which in turn results in the development of disease. As an example, Dr. J. Brailsford wrote of neuralgias of the trunk resulting from compression of nerves "where they traverse bony canals." Dr. A. Oppenheimer noted "narrowing of cervical invertebral foramina" in 66 patients with a wide variety of symptoms. The sensory roots "may be pressed upon by various bones" at the foramina, wrote Dr. C. B. Chamberlain. *Pressure on the spinal nerves, compression . . . in the invertebral foramina, mechanical nerve irritation, "strangling" certain spinal nerves at their exit from the spine,* and *disturbances in the spinal nerves* are a few of the phrases that began to appear in a multitude of medical articles and textbooks and which completely supported chiropractic principles.

And as indication of growing realization of the frequency with which subluxations occur and the seemingly minor forces which in some instances bring them about, a great number of medical doctors mentioned subluxations as having been caused by such commonplace acts as turning the head or sitting up in bed.

Thus, from medicine's own literature, the soundness of chiropractic was demonstrated. It might have seemed logical for the M.D.'s to develop techniques comparable to those of the chiropractors. This, however, has not been the case. Medicine has consistently lagged behind chiropractic and continues to do so today in the field of spinal adjustment, not only because the medical profession places its chief reliance on drug therapy but also because manipulation is, in a sense, merely a "sideline" with most medical doctors while it is the basic therapy of chiropractors. There are medical specialists of many varieties ranging from eye through heart specialists and obstetricians to surgeons who operate in only one area of the body. By the same token, if the overall art of healing is considered, basically, to be a single field with many branches and subdivisions within those branches, then it is obvious why the chiropractor is more competent than the M.D. in the specialty of spinal analysis and adjustment. As a whole, medicine has not accepted the implications of the statement in the *Baruch Report* that ". . . medicine based exclusively on empirical use of pills and potions is becoming obsolete."

The medical trend today, in fact, is toward greater and greater use of "miracle drugs" and vaccines. Numerous types of physical therapy are advocated by the *Baruch Report*—including "the employment of the physical and other effective properties of light, heat, cold, water, electricity, massage, manipulation, exercise, and mechanical devices . . ." Practically all of these methods have been condemned out of hand many times over by organized medicine.

"Physical agents," states the *Baruch Report*, "produce striking biologic responses, including effects on psychic reactions more potent than the effects of many of the drugs gathered through centuries of trial and error . . . The manner in which we use the hospitals and medical schools of today will largely determine the medical future of our country . . ."

The importance of the *Baruch Report* cannot be overestimated. It was one of the most comprehensive studies of so-called "irregular" methods of healing ever undertaken and it cost more than one million dollars. Hundreds of leading scientists participated in gathering information and preparing recommendations.

Regarding medical shortcomings in all aspects of physical therapy and in particular in the field of manipulation, the *Baruch Report* had plenty to say. It asserted that until recently (1944) there had been "little basic or fundamental research" in physical medicine. It stated that the general neglect of physical therapy in the curricula of our medical schools had resulted "in diverting this enormously valuable branch of therapeutics to irregular cults." It expressed the hope that "changes in the medical curriculum now envisioned will constitute the beginnings of a return to the basic principles of the healing art; namely, to treat the patient and not the disease."

This was pulling no punches. The *Report* went on to recommend the establishment of a center of physical medicine in one of the larger medical schools which would "place major emphasis on problems of the structural mechanics of the human body." It warned that there was "a definite need for careful study of the various manipulative procedures which are employed therapeutically to alter the structural mechanics of the human body." And it urged that manipulative therapy be taught in all medical schools of the United States.

Chiropractors would have given blanket endorsement to all this, except for the fact that the *Report* was ideologically eye to eye with organized medicine insofar as maintaining or attaining organized medicine's goal of monopoly of all methods of healing was concerned. It spoke, for example, of nonmedical healers as "irregulars" while advocating medical adoption of their methods. It failed to mention chiropractic or chiropractors, although chiropractic is a legally recognized healing art in the overwhelming majority of the States of the United States; it spoke merely of manipulation in general terms. It recommended the training of many more "well qualified physical therapy technicians" who would work under the direction and supervision of medical doctors; thus it relegated physical therapy to the position of a subordinate branch of healing, like nursing. Its entire "slant" was in the direction of warning the medical doctors to wake up and become as proficient in "irregular" methods of healing as the irregulars were, so that these healing arts would be taken over and absorbed by the medical monopoly and would not develop independently of medicine.

This attitude was not surprising, since many of those who were influential in the planning of the investigation and preparation of the *Report* were leaders in organized medicine. They were not concerned with the development of new methods of healing which would compete on equal terms with medicine; rather they were concerned with preventing the development of these methods except when they were under the aegis of organized medicine.

The *Baruch Report* did not mention that chiropractic was not only the second largest healing art in the world but was also, in most places, as firmly established legislatively as medicine. The use of the blanket term "cults" to define and lump together all the "irregular" healing arts also tended to belittle chiropractic in the minds of those who had heard of it and knew that it was a form of physical therapy but did not know exactly what it was or the high educational requirements of its practitioners.

Following the *Report* the public was given proof of the overwhelming superiority of chiropractic to any form of spinal manipulation taught in the medical schools. The facts were revealed in this way: a letter was sent to the deans of the nation's medical schools inquiring the extent of their teaching of physical medicine to undergraduate medical students. The indifference—or at least the apathy—revealed in regard to the new methods of healing was amazing.

For instance, almost all of the deans admitted that in their schools physical medicine was neglected woefully. A typical admission was to the effect that instruction "up to the present time has been most inadequate." Another stated that "sixteen class hours" were devoted to the subject, another mentioned a course of 126 hours. Still another wrote that his school's course had been "nothing to brag about." And still another admitted that, "This branch of instruction has been sadly neglected, and this neglect is in part responsible for the cults and for a woeful lack of appreciation of its importance by the general practitioner."

The A.M.A. belatedly recognized physical medicine as a specialty within the all-encompassing field of medicine and established a special Section on Physical

Medicine and Rehabilitation. One of the first activities of the new section was to send a questionnaire to the deans of the nation's medical schools, inquiring the status of physical medicine and rehabilitation in their institutions. There were 67 replies, which indicated that, while progress had been made, physical medicine was still a nonentity or a stepchild insofar as many of the medical schools were concerned.

Ten medical schools, for example, did not even have departments of physical education and rehabilitation and were not particularly interested in entering the field. Another 14 were thinking about teaching physio-therapy but had done nothing concrete so far. Another 19 taught physio-therapy as a sideline course. Another 14 had separate departments of physio-therapy, but the course was still very much an adjunct to the instruction in drug therapy. Seventeen offered graduate courses, of short duration, to interested M.D.'s. Forty-five taught undergraduate courses, again short. Thirty-seven taught the subject as a major and graduated students as physio-therapists qualified to work *under medical direction and supervision.*

Contrast this meagre education in not only a sort of manipulation but also a wide variety of other healing methods ranging from the use of light through the employment of mechanical devices—a veritable hodge-podge of sketchy skills—with the chiropractor's thorough education. Not only does the chiropractor study the same basic sciences as the M.D., but his chiropractic subjects (in accredited schools) total 1580 hours. His specific chiropractic subjects are palpation, spinal analysis, clinical instruction, chiropractic principles, X-ray interpretation and nerve tracing.

Chiropractors feel strongly that over the past six decades they have built steadily and surely on a sound theoretical foundation, and have accumulated a body of specialized knowledge and skills which medicine cannot even begin to approach. In the light of the evidence—millions of patients whom chiropractic has cured after medicine, including so-called "physical therapy," has failed—there appears to be ample reason for their confidence.

CHAPTER NINETEEN

Today's Chiropractor

One of the country's leading independent research organizations, the non-profit Public Affairs Institute, has published a study on the modern chiropractor which terms his role in healing the sick as "both large and growing in importance."

The study, "The Present Day Doctor of Chiropractic," was written by Dewey Anderson, Ph.D., Executive Director of the Institute, which publishes research studies on a variety of topics. (It can be obtained, at 25¢ per copy, from the Public Affairs Institute, 312 Pennsylvania Avenue, S.E., Washington 3, D.C.) Dr. Anderson investigated the history and practice of chiropractic, the education of today's chiropractors, the scientific and theoretical foundations of chiropractic, and the criticism of the chiropractic profession by organized medical interests, and covered these topics exhaustively in his 30-page booklet.

Since this was the first time that an independent and unbiased study of the chiropractic profession has been published, the author's findings are of great interest not only to chiropractors but to the public at large.

To Dr. Anderson, the training and habits of mind of today's chiropractor "force him to consider the whole patient, starting with the diagnosis of his problems and going on to their solution—the health of the patient—with care and concern which, while professional in the best sense of that term, is also friendly and cooperative."

The average person, the author states, goes through life with few complicated diseases. But, he adds, we do need more often the attention of trained scientists who can ease our pains, catch troubles before they weaken us, and keep us strong and alert.

"The present day doctor of chiropractic," Dr. Anderson says, "is equipped both by training and experience to treat successfully many of the ills besetting mankind." And he adds, "The role of the trained doctor of chiropractic in helping us overcome bodily pains and ills is therefore both large and growing in importance. He stands in the front line of defense, ready to detect by careful diagnosis any trouble while it's still small and manageable. He is quick to give treatments that relieve pain and suffering. His treatments are intended to send you back to your home or your job fit to work or play and ready to meet life's demands with a serene mind and strong body."

Dr. Anderson explains that chiropractic is a system of treatment and healing "premised on the theories that much disease is caused by interference with the function of the nervous system; that structural maladjustments which cause nerve irritation and lower body resistance are a common though not exclusive cause of disease."

He relates how D. D. Palmer almost 67 years ago

made the discovery of the relationship between the sound functioning of the nervous system and the spinal adjustment, or manipulation. He concludes: "Here is a broadly based system of healing, having its roots in ancient wisdom, tempered by modern scientific discovery and applied with the understanding gained through modern education and training under expert supervision."

A solid scientific and applied training gives the modern doctor of chiropractic the foundation for his special techniques, Dr. Anderson states. He stresses that the chiropractor has had 4,000 class hours of professional education to train him properly in the diagnosis and treatment of disease.

"There is no more chance of the present-day doctor of chiropractic going ahead to treat a new patient in some careless approach to his or her health problem than there is of any other practitioner of any of the healing arts doing so. For professionally he is not only trained to make a careful diagnosis but the success of his treatment depends on the correctness of that diagnosis. What is that treatment which has caused the number of patients seeking chiropractic care to soar so rapidly?

"As simply as a lay person can put the matter, while at the same time seeking to keep entirely within the bounds of known scientific facts, the major emphasis of a chiropractic treatment of the spinal area rests on a manual adjustment and manipulation of the affected area by a doctor qualified to make this adjustment . . .

"Probably none of the other healing arts is better equipped to follow its patients through their daily lives on a continuing and constructive basis than is chiropractic. The sick person visits his doctor of medicine when he is so sick that he just must get relief, or when his fear mounts to the point that he cannot avoid his doctor. But he stays away from that doctor as long as he can, just as he shuns his dentist until a tooth needs pulling.

"Not so with respect to the doctor of chiropractic, for by its very nature a chiropractic treatment is satisfying to the patient and is looked forward to with pleasant anticipation. The chiropractic treatment is so helpful that many people engage their doctor for regular treatments, a system that may add years of helpful, zestful living to their lives.

"The present-day doctor of chiropractic does not regard himself as qualified either by training or experience to treat every condition he meets. He does not seek to practice internal medicine or surgery. But, he is on good terms with specialists who can and do so, to whom he makes referrals of patients. He is in a unique position to form one of a team, offering specialized treatment when that is necessary or desirable to serve the needs of ill people, or to meet the requirements of a community for health services.

"In fact, group practice and team activity in which the several healing arts combine their specialties is increasing, so that it is growing more usual to find a doctor of chiropractic on an industrial staff working alongside the doctor of medicine to keep employees fit; a doctor of chiropractic as part of the health team in a public facility; a doctor of chiropractic on a community health and welfare committee. For the particular value of the trained and experienced chiropractor is becoming recognized at its face value."

Since every profession is built upon a body of knowledge which has developed over a period of years, Dr. Anderson correctly appraises chiropractic in the light of certain concepts which are regarded as well as accepted by the public at large. What about germs, for instance, and the theory that it is germs which cause disease? On this point, Dr. Anderson says:

"Today's chiropractor explains his attitude toward bacteriology and immunology—the germ theory of disease—as follows: Of course bacteria and viruses can cause disease, and do. But the extent to which they successfully attack the human body depends upon the level of resistance of the body. The role of the nervous system in establishing and maintaining body strength or building up resistance after infection has taken hold must not be discounted. Hence, the present-day chiropractor's ability to improve body tone through the correction or lessening of nerve irritation and prescription of hygienic practices and good nursing care become important factors in the cure of disease.

"From a handful of patients somewhat more than half a century ago who came to D. D. Palmer (chiropractic's discoverer) and got relief, those being cared for by today's chiropractors number many millions. And every year the number swells as chiropractors become more proficient and as their satisfied and healthy patients spread the word. Here is the best and final test of an emerging profession seriously serving the public."

Dr. Anderson relates the history of professional education in the United States and recalls the days, some 44 years ago, when medical education in this country was condemned as a hazard to the sick. He points out that standards are constantly improving in all fields.

207

"Today," he says, "the graduate of an accredited chiropractic college is as well qualified to practice his healing art as the graduate of an accredited medical college is qualified to practice medicine as his form of the healing art. Often, too, they both have to pass the same state board examinations in the basic sciences to obtain a license.

"During his four years of training, the present-day doctor of chiropractic takes 740 hours of instruction and laboratory work in anatomy, including embryology and histology; 240 hours of physiology; 180 hours of biochemistry; 520 hours of pathology and bacteriology; 200 hours of obstetrics and gynecology; and 1,960 hours of diagnosis and treatment following the special principles of his healing art, covering such subjects as neurology, pediatrics, dermatology and roentgenology.

"The present-day doctor of chiropractic is not only well equipped in the basic sciences, classroom and laboratory study of his profession, but undergoes many hours of practice under supervision before being graduated. This is the counterpart of what happens with the medical students who must depend on hospital internships for their bedside training, a projection into the modern day of the apprentice system which has proved so invaluable in providing competency. In addition, the more advanced training centers have added clinical training and strong pressure is underway to admit chiropractors to service in public and veterans' hospitals.

"All these advances have strengthened the professional position and opportunities for service of present-day doctors of chiropractic. The insurance companies have responded to this situation, and well over 500 now accept chiropractors' certification on claims. The trend is so pronounced that it is safe to say that these cautious business institutions are universally recognizing the safety, integrity, and professional competence of chiropractors.

"Business and industry have come increasingly to view the chiropractic form of the healing art as helpful in keeping workers fit. Thus the nationally operated Western Union Telegraph Company assures that chiropractic certification will be accepted for employee benefits.

"Probably in few other groups has chiropractic been so widely and universally acclaimed as in athletics. Professional and amateur athletic organizations have employed staffs of doctors of chiropractic to keep their members fit.

"Chiropractic has proven its worth in the care of veterans. As a result the Veterans of Foreign Wars and the Disabled American Veterans, among other veterans' organizations, have consistently and actively supported chiropractic as a method of healing and urged for it undiscriminating and fair treatment in legislation offered both nationally and in the several states.

"The Chiropractic Research Foundation reports successful treatment of both acute and chronic polio by chiropractic methods.

"Chief among those who testify to their increasingly valuable experiences with the work of doctors of chiropractic are their patients. It is these satisfied patients who tell the story to their neighbors and friends. They defend the profession from unfair attacks. They urge equality of treatment before the laws of the states and nation for this form of the healing art whose effectiveness has been demonstrated in their own cases."

What of the future of chiropractic? Dr. Anderson is well aware that strong attacks have been made on the practice of chiropractic. After examining the nature of these attacks, he says that most practicing medical men have no time to judge its merits and appreciate the fact that such attacks represent the natural antagonism of an existing profession toward a successful newcomer.

Most of the attacks, he points out, are made by "the professional political arm of medicine," and he says, "an unbiased, impartial appraisal of chiropractic is seldom, if ever, forthcoming from such sources."

"In these days of high-speed living, stresses and strains and resultant nerve-exhaustion," says Dr. Anderson, "chiropractic is fast becoming an indispensable element in helping people maintain good health."

He concludes: "For chiropractic science and its application by means of a present-day chiropractor's consultation and treatment, function with the whole man in mind. Starting with the base of neuro-anatomical structure and seeing the man in his daily environment, chiropractic seeks to make a proper alignment between the function of this basic apparatus and nutrition and elimination as basic aspects of the physiological manifestations of living. The training and experience of the doctor of chiropractic equip him particularly well to provide professional advice and treatment where needed in this complex task of adjusting the individual and his surroundings.

"Add to the foregoing the fact that the doctor of

chiropractic is striving to build his profession, to meet his social responsibilities, to take his place as a leader in the community. In this he has developed a code of ethics that manifests high regard for the rights of his patients, a commitment to the 'golden rule' of individual conduct, and a sense that the integrity of his own occupation rests on his recognition of the integrity of every other occupation within the broad field of the healing art.

"The way ahead is becoming clearer with the passage of time. Much of the unreasoned heat has gone out of the opposition of the longer-established medical profession, and the attacks still being made on chiropractic are more tempered. There are a growing number of practitioners of the older forms of the healing art who work alongside the doctors of chiropractic in professional accord, each doing that part of the job of providing health services which his training and experience best qualify him to do. This feature of team work holds great hope for the future, and much good will result for people who need both kinds of care.

"Finally, it can be said in closing this brief description of chiropractic that the profession itself is so ardent about its future that nothing can stop doctors of chiropractic from being devoted public servants and becoming better ones with the passage of time."

CHAPTER TWENTY

The Future—Can Chiropractic Help You?

Can chiropractic help *you?*

The answer to this question is not so simple as it might appear. Chiropractors do not profess to be miracle workers, able to cure anything under the sun. Among the conditions in which chiropractic is of little or no benefit are various hereditary abnormalities such as defective nerve fibers, faulty metabolism, excess cerebro-spinal fluid, or conditions of irreversible pathology. The chiropractic examination, which includes not only standard procedures employed by medical doctors but specialized chiropractic procedures as well, will reveal whether or not these conditions are present.

Then there is a wide area reserved to the medical profession in which chiropractors do not attempt to practice. Although chiropractors deal with structural adjustments, they do not set broken bones; that province is reserved to the medical doctor. Nor do chiropractors treat cuts and wounds, perform surgery, practice obstetrics, or prescribe or administer drugs. When a condition appears to be outside his particular field, the chiropractor refers the patient to a dentist, gynecologist, optometrist, surgeon, syphilogist, etc.

The chiropractor does not profess to be able to help after the disease condition has reached a point where its progress is irreversible, even though the functioning of the nervous system may be restored by chiropractic. He may only be able to alleviate suffering and prolong life. In cases of malignancy in which the prognosis is bad, for example, chiropractic frequently is able to eliminate abnormal afferent or incoming sensory impulses originating in the tumor area and improve general bodily functionings, thus greatly reducing or even eliminating the necessity for taking drugs and opiates and increasing the remaining life expectancy.

It should always be remembered that the chiropractor is a structural engineer of the body, a "bio-engineer" as contrasted with the drug practitioner, who is a "biochemist." More properly, he might be termed a "bio-electrical-engineer" since he is concerned with the transmission of electrical impulses via the nerves. It is easy to see why chiropractic has been successful in such a wide variety of ills, which in turn have a wide variety of structural causes. As chiropractic research has demonstrated, there are a multitude of environmental factors which can and do get the body structures out of perfect alignment and as a consequence impair nerve functioning and invite disease. Some of these are:

Faulty posture—the "original sin" in chiropractic thinking. Incidentally, chiropractors, regardless of age, have the best posture of any group in our society, since they know the importance of preventive therapy as well as of corrective therapy.

Falls, blows, strains, jolts and twists. There are few persons who are not subject to these accidents or occupational injuries and to most of us they occur quite frequently. Chiropractors emphasize that a subluxation or other structural misalignment may be no more than microscopic in degree to cause serious derangement of nerve functioning.

Asymmetries due to "lop sided" activities in work or play. These activities tend to strengthen certan muscles at the expense of others and pull the spine out of line. Among such activities are games like bowling, tennis, baseball, and golf, and such work as typing and plastering. (A much more complete list is given in Chapter Four.)

Fatigue. Merely notice how the tired person tends to "droop" and perhaps let his stomach "drop," and the importance of fatigue will become obvious.

Exposure to heat, cold, pain, humidity, and drafts can cause muscular contractions that in turn bring on structural defects. Correction of these defects by the chiropractor frequently results in amazingly swift cure of a multitude of so called "low-resistance" ills such as the common cold, pneumonia, influenza, grippe, sinusitis, and mastoiditis.

Emotion. When a person is disturbed by worry, fear, grief, and other emotions, structural tensions are present. Merely notice the characteristic postures of elation and despair to be convinced of this. Because the chiropractor "cuts through" these tensions and allows the nervous system to function normally again, he often accomplishes remarkable results with the emotionally disturbed. Many ailments, such as peptic ulcer, are known to be of emotional origin; in these, too, the chiropractor is highly successful.

The above is but a partial list of factors which often

result in structural maladjustment and consequent illness. The chiropractor can often detect "short circuits" in the nervous system and microscopic subluxations before symptoms begin to develop; he can therefore prevent disease by making its incubation impossible. For this reason, many prudent patients make periodic visits to their chiropractors as a matter of course just for checkups, on the same principle that many people see their medical doctors or dentists at regular intervals, even when feeling fine.

In Part Two was listed a wide variety of ailments in which chiropractic has proven highly successful, frequently after medical care had failed. In many of these, as proven by comparison of many thousands of medical and chiropractic patients, chiropractic consistently achieves higher percentages of both cure and alleviation, a fact which is all the more remarkable because so many of the patients had turned to chiropractors only after M.D.'s had given them up and their powers of resistance and recuperation were, at best, at very low ebb. The great chiropractic research organizations and associations insist that if all of these patients had come to chiropractors at the commencement of their illnesses, the superiority of chiropractic over medical therapy would be even more strikingly demonstrated.

There is striking evidence that chiropractic not only cures or benefits a higher percentage of patients than do other forms of therapy, but that it achieves these results in shorter time and at less cost; and finally, that the benefits of chiropractic are more lasting. The evidence is to be found in the records of many impartial sources such as accident and health insurance companies, mutual benefit societies and fraternal organizations, unions, state workmen's compensation boards, large industrial plants, and numerous others.

Canada's Foundry Journal reported in its June, 1956, issue the results of an industrial survey from the files of Workmen's Compensation Boards in 44 States of the U.S.A. and in Canada. The survey was limited to a study of low-back injuries treated by three methods, chiropractic, osteopathy, and medicine. In all, 4,746 cases of low-back injuries were included in the survey. Crushing injuries, fractures, and others requiring surgery were not included. The cases treated in hospitals were not considered to be any more serious than those treated outside of hospital.

The *Journal* gives these findings:

"The figures of the greatest significance were probably those dealing with the relative number of work days lost under the different types of care. Medical (non-hospitalized) with 19.9 days, medical (hospitalized) with 33.8 days, osteopathy with 11.5, and chiropractic with 10.9 days off work. Any type of care which results in less time lost means a resulting drop in labour turnover and less re-training. Both are expensive factors in production. For labour this means more take-home pay and new opportunity to regain health rapidly.

"Also of significance are the figures showing the amount of compensation paid in each of the four categories. Since the number of days off work directly affects the amount of compensation, the chiropractic grouping indicates the savings possible when this type of care is employed for such injuries.

The compensation paid was, for the group treated by chiropractic, $27.07; osteopathy, $35.46; medical (non-hospitalized) $50.06; medical (hospitalized), $85.34.

"The wages lost by the worker were reported as follows: chiropractic $55.52; osteopathy $76.06; medical (non-hospitalized) $95.06; medical (hospitalized) $163.44. The average cost of professional care in the four groups was: chiropractic $27.88; osteopathy $29.85; medical (non-hospitalized) $27.07; medical (hospitalized) $121.45. These figures do not show the same great difference in cost, but coupled to the great savings shown by the previous statistics the total cost of chiropractic care reveals a significant saving for the worker, the Compensation Board, and the industry; not only in money but also in man-hours. The total cost table shows the following figures: chiropractic $56.12; osteopathy $64.19; medical (non-hospitalized) $67.69; medical (hospitalized) $209.48."

Canada's Foundry Journal makes this conclusion: "Spinal injuries are one of the commonest causes of time-loss and pay-loss in industry. This is especially true, of course, in heavy industry . . . The results of this survey proved conclusively that chiropractic care of low-back injuries has no equal and can be of tremendous benefit in reducing the lost man-hours and lost wages suffered by those afflicted with this painful condition."

Medical Economics noted in its advice to the medical profession:

"Do you think the average American is too ignorant

to know what's good for him? If not, why not let him decide whether he wants to go to a chiropractor? . . . The chiropractors assure us that they don't in any way want to restrict doctors of medicine. Why, then, should you seek to restrict *them*? They'll concede that there's something in medicine and surgery. Why won't you concede that there may be something in chiropractic? What's fair for one, is fair for the other. Isn't that the American way?"

Indeed that is the American way—the right of free choice after examination of the facts. This right is, of course, explicitly guaranteed in the Constitution of the United States. Every American has the right to choose his doctor and whatever type of therapy that doctor may employ.

The question is not whether one should give up the services of a medical doctor and entrust himself exclusively to a chiropractor. Each has his clearly defined place in the great complex of the over-all art of healing. Each may, in many an instance, complement the other to the benefit of the patient whom both are trying to aid.

Chiropractic's unique contribution toward eliminating a wide number of ailments has been growing despite the obstacles presented by special interest groups. In the years ahead, chiropractic is destined to serve an ever increasing number of people—and from all indications, serve them well!

Appendices

The Year the Chiropractic Act Was Passed in Each State and Province of Canada

Alabama	1959	North Carolina	1917
Arizona	1921	North Dakota	1913
Arkansas	1915	Ohio	1915
California	1922	Oklahoma	1921
Colorado	1933	Oregon	1915
Connecticut	1917	Pennsylvania	1951
Delaware	1937	Rhode Island	1923
District of Columbia	1929	South Carolina	1932
Florida	1919	South Dakota	1921
Georgia	1921	Tennessee	1923
Idaho	1919	Texas	1949
Illinois	1923	Utah	1923
Indiana	1927	Vermont	1919
Iowa	1921	Virginia	1944
Kansas	1913	Washington	1919
Kentucky	1928	West Virginia	1925
Maine	1924	Wisconsin	1925
Maryland	1929	Wyoming	1929
Michigan	1933	Alaska	1939
Minnesota	1919	Hawaii	1925
Missouri	1927	Puerto Rico	1952
Montana	1918	Alberta	1923
Nebraska	1916	British Columbia	1934
Nevada	1923	Manitoba	1945
New Hampshire	1921	New Brunswick	1958
New Jersey	1953	Ontario	1925
New Mexico	1921	Saskatchewan	1943

APPENDIX B

Chiropractic Boards of Examiners in the United States and Canada

Below is a list of the secretaries of each Board and the educational requirements for a State Chiropractic License.

Note: Members of the State Boards of Chiropractic Examiners are officially appointed by the governors of the various jurisdictions.

ALABAMA

Secretary: R. R. Williamson, D.C., 200 W. Point Street, Roanoke.

Educational Requirements: Four-year standard chiropractic college course, Basic Science Certificate.

ALASKA

Secretary: B. W. Steele, D.C., 509 Fireweed, Anchorage.

Educational Requirements: Two years of liberal arts college, 4 years of 9 months (4000 hours) of chiropractic college, Alaska Basic Science Certificate.

ARIZONA

Secretary: Vernon P. Pierce, D.C., Box 1751, Miami.

Educational Requirements: Four years of chiropractic college of not less than 9 months each.

ARKANSAS

Secretary: A. H. Swain, D.C., 404 S.W. Avenue, El Dorado.

Educational Requirements: Chiropractic college course of 4 years of 9 months each (3600 hours), Basic Science Certificate.

CALIFORNIA

Secretary: Westley E. Rodgers, D.C., 151 College Avenue, Santa Rosa.

Educational Requirements: Chiropractic college course of 4 years of 9 months each (4000 hours), 2 years of liberal arts college.

COLORADO

Secretary: Leo E. Wunsch, D.C., 1601 Vine, Denver.

Educational Requirements: Chiropractic college course of 4 years (4000 hours), Basic Science Certificate.

CONNECTICUT

Secretary: Harry Sprovireo, D.C., 1188 Main Street, Bridgeport.

Educational Requirements: Two years of liberal arts college, chiropractic college course of 4 years of 8 months each (4000 hours), Basic Science Certificate.

DELAWARE

Secretary: Frank Goble, 104 S. Bradford Street, Dover.

Educational Requirements: Two years of liberal arts college, chiropractic college course of 4 years of 8 months each.

DISTRICT OF COLUMBIA

Secretary: William S. Lineweaver, D.C., 1025 Connecticut Avenue, N.W.

Educational Requirements: Two years of liberal arts college, chiropractic college course of 4 years of 9 months each, Basic Science Certificate.

FLORIDA

Secretary: D. I. Rainey, D.C., Box 231, Tallahassee.

Educational Requirements: Chiropractic college course of 4 years (4000 hours), Basic Science Certificate.

GEORGIA

Secretary: C. L. Clifton, 224 Capitol, Atlanta.

Educational Requirements: One year of liberal arts college, chiropractic college course of 4 years of 9 months each.

HAWAII

Secretary: Donald T. L. Ching, D.C., 1136–12th Avenue, Honolulu.

Educational Requirements: Two years of liberal arts college, chiropractic college course of 4 years of 9 months each (4200 hours).

IDAHO

Secretary: H. R. Walmsely, D.C., 1615—4th Street S., Nampa.

Educational Requirements: Two years of liberal arts college, chiropractic college course of 4 years of 8 months each.

ILLINOIS

Secretary: L. P. Rehberger, D.C., Highland.

Educational Requirements: Chiropractic college course of 4 years of 8 months each.

Appendix B

INDIANA
Secretary: Clarence F. Aumann, D.C., 326 North Emerson Avenue, Indianapolis.
Educational Requirements: Two years of liberal arts college, chiropractic college course of 4 years (4000 hours).

IOWA
Secretary: H. T. Opsahl, D.C., Chiropractic Division, State House, Des Moines.
Educational Requirements: Chiropractic college course of 4 years (4000 hours), Basic Science Certificate.

KANSAS
Secretary: Dean L. Wise, D.C., 1601 S. Water, Wichita.
Educational Requirements: Approved chiropractic college course of 4 years of 9 months each, Basic Science Certificate.

KENTUCKY
Secretary: J. N. Riggs, D.C., 2021 W. Jefferson Street, Louisville.
Educational Requirements: Approved chiropractic college course of 4 years of 9 months each (4000 hours).

MAINE
Secretary: H. M. Burry, D.C., Main Street, Milo.
Educational Requirements: Two years of liberal arts college, chiropractic college course of 4 years (4400 hours).

MARYLAND
Secretary: Adam Baer, D.C., 22 Broadway, Frostburg.

Educational Requirements: Two years of liberal arts college, chiropractic college course of 4 years (4000 hours).

MICHIGAN

Secretary: Charles C. Lynch, D.C., 2208 W. Grand Boulevard, Detroit.

Educational Requirements: Chiropractic college course of 4 years 9 months each (4000 hours), Basic Science Certificate.

MINNESOTA

Secretary: Victor L. Marty, D.C., 2903 E. 42nd Street, Minneapolis.

Educational Requirements: Chiropractic college course of 4 years of 8 months each (4000 hours), Basic Science Certificate.

MISSOURI

Secretary: S. J. Durham, D.C., 204½ E. High Street, Jefferson City.

Educational Requirements: Chiropractic college course.

MONTANA

Secretary: M. J. Klette, D.C., Box 709, Havre.

Educational Requirements: Two years of liberal arts college, chiropractic college course of 4 years of 9 months each.

NEBRASKA

Secretary: M. B. DeJarnette, D.C., P.O. Box 1164, Nebraska City.

Educational Requirements: Chiropractic college course of 4 years of 9 months each (4000 hours), Basic Science Certificate.

NEVADA
Secretary: Robert W. Warburton, D.C., 329 N. Sierra Street, Reno.
Educational Requirements: Chiropractic college course of 4 years (4000 hours), Basic Science Certificate.

NEW HAMPSHIRE
Secretary: Max Winer, D.C., Morrill Building, Dover.
Educational Requirements: Chiropractic college course of 4 years (4000 hours).

NEW JERSEY
Secretary: Cecil L. Martin, D.C., 3630 Hudson Boulevard, Jersey City.
Educational Requirements: Two years of liberal arts college, chiropractic college course of 4 years of 9 months each.

NEW MEXICO
Secretary: H. D. Shaw, D.C., 4508 Fourth Street N.W., Albuquerque.
Educational Requirements: Chiropractic college course of 4 years (4000 hours).

NORTH CAROLINA
Secretary: Carl H. Peters, D.C., 119 Coast Line Street, Rocky Mount.
Educational Requirements: Two years of liberal arts college, chiropractic college course of 4 years of 9 months each.

NORTH DAKOTA
Secretary: J. W. Payne, D.C., Box 619, Williston.

Educational Requirements: Two years of liberal arts college, chiropractic college course.

OHIO

Secretary: Fred M. MacLean, D.C., 48 E. Liberty Street, Girard.

Educational Requirements: Two years of liberal arts college, chiropractic college course.

OKLAHOMA

Secretary: R. V. Heinze, D.C., 117 E. Cleveland, Mangum.

Educational Requirements: Two years of liberal arts college, chiropractic college course of 4 years of 9 months each (4,150 hours), Basic Science Certificate.

OREGON

Secretary: Anton Latham, D.C., 3905 S.E. Belmont Street, Portland.

Educational Requirements: Two years of liberal arts college, chiropractic college course of 4 years of 9 months each (4000 hours), Basic Science Certificate.

PENNSYLVANIA

Secretary: Mrs. Emily L. Garberich, Box 911, Harrisburg.

Educational Requirements: One year of college sciences, chiropractic college course of 4 years of 9 months each (4000 hours).

PUERTO RICO

Secretary: Herminio Mendez Herrera, Box 9222, Santurce.

Educational Requirements: Two years of liberal arts

college, chiropractic college course of 4 years
(4000 hours).

RHODE ISLAND
Secretary: W. A. Watkinson, D.C., 372 Broadway,
Newport.
Educational Requirements: One year of liberal arts
college, chiropractic college course of 4 years of
8 months each, Basic Science Certificate.

SOUTH CAROLINA
Secretary: F. Chas. Holliday, D.C., 421 West Meeting
Street, Lancaster.
Educational Requirements: Chiropractic college course
of 4 years of 9 months each.

SOUTH DAKOTA
Secretary: D. R. McDowell, D.C., 122 W. 10th, Sioux
Falls.
Educational Requirements: Chiropractic college course
of 4 years of 9 months each, Basic Science Cer-
tificate.

TENNESSEE
Secretary: J. W. Lawrence, D.C., West End Heights,
Lebanon.
Educational Requirements: Chiropractic college course
of 4 years of 9 months each, Basic Science Cer-
tificate.

TEXAS
Secretary: Charles E. Courtion, D.C., 305 West
Concho, San Angelo.
Educational Requirements: 120 semester hours of col-
lege—acceptable to the University of Texas for

a B.A. degree, chiropractic college course of 4 years of 8 months each, Basic Science Certificate.

UTAH

Secretary: B. Keith Benner, D.C., 38 East 4th South, Bountiful.

Educational Requirements: One year liberal arts college, chiropractic college course of 4 years of 9 months each (4000 hours).

VERMONT

Secretary: Richard T. Smith. D.C., 146 Main Street, Montpelier.

Educational Requirements: Chiropractic college course of 4 years of 9 months each (4400 hours).

VIRGINIA

Secretary: H. H. Dodge, D.C., Central National Bank Building, Richmond.

Educational Requirements: Two years liberal arts college, chiropractic college course of 4 years of 8 months each.

WASHINGTON

Secretary: John Pettersen, D.C., 1808 Seventh Avenue, Seattle.

Educational Requirements: Chiropractic college course of 4 years (4000 hours).

WEST VIRGINIA

Secretary: R. E. Tripp, D.C., 409 Professional Bldg., Fairmont.

Educational Requirements: Two years of liberal arts college, chiropractic college course of 4 years of 9 months each (4000 hours).

Appendix B

WISCONSIN
  Secretary: S. C. Syverud, D.C., 320 West Main Street, Mount Horeb.
  Educational Requirements: Two years of liberal arts college, chiropractic college course of 4 years of 9 months each (3600 hours), Basic Science Certificate.

WYOMING
  Secretary: Gordon L. Holman, D.C., 2811 Central Avenue, Cheyenne.
  Educational Requirements: Two years of liberal arts college, chiropractic college course of 4 years of 9 months each (4000 hours).

DOMINION OF CANADA

ALBERTA
  Secretary: J. C. Speelman, D.C., 511–7th Street So., Lethbridge.
  Educational Requirements: Junior matriculation, chiropractic college course of 4 years of 8 months each.

BRITISH COLUMBIA
  Secretary: B. A. Evans, D.C., 6449 Royal Oak Avenue, South Burnaby.
  Educational Requirements: Junior matriculation, chiropractic college course of 4 years of 8 months each.

NEW BRUNSWICK
  Secretary: Robert Randall, D.C., 126 Steadman Street, Moncton, N.B.

Educational Requirements: Senior matriculation, chiropractic college course of 4 years of 9 months each.

MANITOBA

Secretary: J. D. Mowat, D.C., 204 Norlyn Building, Winnipeg.

Educational Requirements: Junior matriculation, chiropractic college course of 4 academic years.

ONTARIO

Secretary: James W. Ellison, D.C., 102 Annette Street, Toronto.

Educational Requirements: Junior matriculation, chiropractic college course of 4 years of 9 months each (4200 hours).

SASKATCHEWAN

Secretary: N. K. Cram, University of Saskatchewan, Saskatoon.

Educational Requirements: Junior matriculation, chiropractic college course of 4 years of 8 months each.

Note: Chiropractic is not regulated in Louisiana, Massachusetts, Mississippi, New York, and the Province of Quebec, at the present writing.

APPENDIX C

*List and Classification of
Insurance Companies
Granting Recognition to the
Chiropractic Profession*

**Insurance Companies Approved by the Chiropractic
Profession As Granting Comprehensive Coverage**
This classification lists some 600 companies which are
approved as providing comprehensive coverage, which
includes chiropractic care. Nearly 100 other companies
offering limited chiropractic recognition are classified as
B companies and are not listed herein.

Class "A-1"—Includes insurance companies which
grant full recognition to chiropractic by specifically stating
in their policies that policyholders may have necessary
chiropractic treatment on the same basis as medical treatment.

Class "A"—Includes insurance companies which ap-
prove chiropractic services for their policyholders or in-
sureds and pay legitimate chiropractic claims but do not
so indicate in all of their policies.

Companies Classified A-1
Accident Indemnity Insurance Co., Greensboro, N. C.
American Aviation & General Ins. Co., Reading, Pa.
American Bankers Insurance Co., Charlotte, N. C.
American Benefit Association, Minneapolis, Minn.
American Casualty Company, Reading, Pa.
American Farmers Insurance Company, Phoenix, Ariz.

American Life and Accident Insurance Co., St. Louis, Mo.
American Life & Casualty Insurance Co., Fargo, N. D.
American Mutual Liability Insurance Co., Boston, Mass.
American & Southern Ins. Co., Greensboro, N. C.
Atlantic & Pacific Insurance Co., Denver, Colo.
Atlas Mutual Life Insurance Company, Indianapolis, Ind.
Auto-Owners Insurance Company, Lansing, Michigan
Canada Health & Accident Insurance Co., Waterloo, Ont.
Central Assurance Co., Columbus, Ohio
Central National Life Insurance Co., Jacksonville, Ill.
Central Standard Life Insurance Company, Chicago, Ill.
Combined American Insurance Company, Dallas, Texas
Commercial Travelers Mutual Accident Ass'n of America,
    Utica, New York
Dixie Life & Accident Insurance Co., Little Rock, Ark.
Eastern Cross Insurance Co., Charlotte, N. C.
Employees Mutual Benefit Association, St. Paul, Minn.
Fidelity Reserve Insurance Company, Little Rock, Ark.
First National Casualty Company, Fond du Lac, Wis.
Globe Life & Accident Ins. Co., Oklahoma City, Okla.
Golden State Mutual Life Insurance Co., Los Angeles,
    Calif.
Great Eastern Mutual Life Insurance Co., Denver, Colo.
Great Southern Life Insurance Co., Houston, Texas
Illinois Mutual Casualty Company, Peoria, Illinois
Interstate Assurance Company, Des Moines, Iowa
Iowa Hardware Mutual Insurance Co., Mason City, Iowa
Iowa Home Mutual Casualty Co., Des Moines, Iowa
Manufacturers & Merchants Indemnity Co., Cincinnati,
    Ohio
Minnesota Commercial Men's Association, Minneapolis,
    Minnesota
Missouri National Life Insurance Co., Kansas City, Mo.
Mutual Benefit Health & Accident Assn., Omaha, Nebr.
Mutual Creamery Insurance Company, Cottonwood,
    Minn.

Mutual Life Underwriters, Doland, S. D.
Mutual Protective Ins. Co., Omaha, Nebr.
National Indemnity Company, Omaha, Nebr.
Northern Security life Insurance Company, Aurora, Ill.
Old Equity Life Ins. Co., Evanston, Ill.
Old Security Life Insurance Co., Kansas City, Mo.
Olympic National Life Insurance Co., Seattle, Wash.
Pennsylvania Life Insurance Co., Los Angeles, Calif.
Peoples Accident Insurance Company, Lincoln, Nebr.
Prudence Life Insurance Co., Chicago, Ill.
Security National Life Insurance Co., St. Louis, Mo.
S. D. Benevolent Society, Doland, S. D.
Southern States Life Insurance Co., Houston, Texas
Sovereign States Insurance Co., Nashville, Tenn.
The Union Labor Life Insurance Co., New York, N. Y.
United Benefit Life Insurance Company, Omaha, Nebr.
United Insurance Co. of America, Chicago, Ill.
Valley Forge Insurance Co., Reading, Pa.
Valley Forge Life Insurance Co., Reading, Pa.
Washington National Life Insurance Co., Evanston, Ill.
Western Mutual Life & Casualty Co., Rapid City, S. D.
World Insurance Company, Omaha, Nebr.

Companies Classified A

Acacia Mutual Life Insurance Co., Washington, D. C.
Accident & Casualty Insurance Co., New York, N. Y.
Accident Fire & Life Corp., Philadelphia, Pa.
Aetna Casualty & Surety Company, Hartford, Conn.
Aetna Insurance Co., Hartford, Conn.
Aetna Life Insurance Company, Hartford, Conn.
Agricultural Life Insurance Company, Detroit, Mich.
All American Life & Casualty Co., Park Ridge, Ill.
Alliance Casualty Company, Philadelphia, Pa.
Alliance Mutual Casualty Company, McPherson, Kan.
Allied Mutual Casualty Company, Des Moines, Iowa
Allstate Insurance Company, Chicago, Illinois

Amalgamated Labor Life Insurance Co. of Florida, Miami, Fla.
American Associated Insurance Co., St. Louis, Mo.
American Automobile Insurance Co., St. Louis, Mo.
American Employers Insurance Co., Boston, Mass.
American Family Life Insurance Co., Columbus, Ga.
American Fidelity & Casualty Co., Inc., Richmond, Va.
American Guarantee & Liability Ins. Co., Chicago, Ill.
American Health Insurance Corp., Baltimore, Maryland
American Heritage Life Insurance Co., Jacksonville, Fla.
American Home Assurance Co., New York, N. Y.
American Independent Mutual Casualty Co., Philadelphia, Pa.
American Liability & Surety Company, Cincinnati, O.
American Life & Accident Ins. Co. of Kentucky, Louisville, Ky.
American Manufacturers Mutual Insurance Co., Chicago, Ill.
American Motorists, Chicago, Illinois
American Mutual Life Insurance Co., Des Moines, Iowa
American National Insurance Co., Galveston, Texas
American Policy Holders Insurance Co., Boston, Mass.
American Protective Health & Accident Co., Lincoln, Nebr.
American Republic Insurance Co. Des Moines, Iowa
American Reserve Life Insurance Co., Omaha, Nebr.
American States Insurance Company, Indianapolis, Ind.
American Surety Company of New York, New York, N. Y.
American Travelers Association, Indianapolis, Ind.
American Underwriters Health & Accident Ins. Co., Peoria, Illinois
American United Life Insurance Co., Indianapolis, Ind.
Anchor Casualty Company, St. Paul, Minn.
Atlantic Life Insurance Company, Richmond, Va.
Atlantic Mutual Insurance Co., New York, N. Y.
Automobile Casualty Insurance Co., Los Angeles, Calif.

Automobile Dealers Mutual Insurance Co., Kansas City, Mo.

Automobile Mutual Insurance Company of America, Providence, Rhode Island

Babcock Co., A. H. Agents, Loraine, Ohio

Bankers Casualty Company, Minneapolis, Minn.

Bankers Health & Accident Company, Houston, Texas

Bankers Indemnity Insurance Co., Newark, N. J.

Bankers Life & Casualty Co., Chicago, Ill.

Bankers Life and Loan Company, Dallas, Texas

Bankers Life Company, Des Moines, Iowa

Bankers National Life Ins. Co., Montclair, N. J.

Bankers Union Life Insurance Company, Denver, Colo.

Beacon Mutual Indemnity Company, Columbus, Ohio

Beneficial Casualty Insurance Co., Los Angeles, Calif.

Bituminous Casualty Corp., Rock Island, Ill.

Boston Insurance Co., Boston, Mass.

Brotherhood Accident Company, Boston, Mass.

Brotherhood of Locomotive Engineers, U. S. A.

Brotherhood of Railway Trainmen, U. S. A.

Buckeye Mutual Accident Ass'n, Toledo, Ohio

Buckeye Union Casualty Co., Columbus, Ohio

Business Men's Accident Association of America, Phila., Pa.

Business Men's Assurance Company of America, Kansas City, Mo.

Business Men's Insurance Co., Greensboro, N. C.

Business Men's Insurance Company, Kansas City, Mo.

Business Men's Protective Ass'n, Des Moines, Iowa

California Casualty Indemnity Exchange, San Francisco, Calif.

California Insurance Co., New York, N. Y.

Canadian Order of Woodmen of World, London, Ont., Can.

Car & General Ins. Corp., Ltd., London, England

Catholic Knights of St. George, Pittsburgh, Pa.

Catholic Ladies of Columbia, Columbus, Ohio
Celina Mutual Casualty Company, Celina, Ohio
Central Life Assurance Society, Des Moines, Iowa
Central National Insurance Companies, Omaha, Nebr.
Central States Health & Life Co. of Omaha,
	Omaha, Nebr.
Central Surety & Insurance Corp., Kansas City, Mo.
Checker Mutual Automobile Insurance Co., Detroit, Mich.
Cheese Makers Mutual Casualty Co., Madison, Wis.
Cherokee Credit Life Insurance Co., Macon, Ga.
Chicago Ice Producers Mutual Liability Co., Chicago, Ill.
Citadel Life Insurance Co., Charlotte, N. C.
Citizens Mutual Automobile Insurance Co., Howell, Mich.
Cloverleaf Life & Casualty Co., Jacksonville, Ill.
Coal Operators Casualty Co., Greensburg, Pa.
Coastal Plain Life Insurance Co., Rocky Mount, N. C.
College Life Insurance Co. of America, Indianapolis, Ind.
Colonial Life & Accident Company, Columbia, S. C.
Colorado Credit Life, Boulder, Colo.
Colorado Insurance Group, Boulder, Colo.
Colorado Life Insurance Company, Denver, Colo.
Columbia Casualty Co., New York, New York
Columbian National Life Insurance Co., Boston, Mass.
Columbus Mutual Life Insurance Co., Columbus, Ohio
Combined Insurance Co. of America, Chicago, Ill.
Commercial Accident Company, Springfield, Illinois
Commercial General Insurance Co., Hartford, Conn.
Commercial Insurance Co., Newark, N. J.
Commercial Mutual Insurance Co., Cincinnati, Ohio
Commercial Union Assurance Co., New York, N. Y.
Connecticut General Life Insurance Co., Hartford, Conn.
Connecticut Indemnity Company, New Haven, Conn.
Connecticut Mutual Life Insurance Co., Hartford, Conn.
Consolidated Casualty Insurance Co., Houston, Texas
Continental Assurance Company, Chicago, Ill.
Continental Casualty Company, Chicago, Ill.

Appendix C

Country Life Insurance Company, Chicago, Illinois
Country Mutual Casualty Company, Chicago, Ill.
Craftsman Insurance Company, Boston, Mass.
Croatian Fraternal Union, Pittsburgh, Pa.
Danes' Brotherhood Camp No. 139, Viborg, N. D.
Dearborn National Insurance Company, Detroit, Mich.
Detroit Automobile Inter-Insurance Exchange, Detroit, Mich.
Detroit Mutual Accident Ins. Co., Detroit, Mich.
Detroit Mutual Automobile Ins. Co., Detroit, Mich.
Detroit Mutual Insurance Company, Detroit, Mich.
Duluth Casualty Company, Duluth, Minn.
Eastern Commercial Travelers Accident Assn., Boston, Mass.
Eastern Commercial Travelers Health Assn., Boston, Mass.
Eastern Mutual Insurance Co., Boston, Massachusetts
Educators Mutual Life Insurance Co., Lancaster, Pa.
Electrical Workers Benefit Association, Washington, District of Columbia
Emmco Casualty Insurance Company, South Bend, Ind.
Empire Life & Accident Company, Indianapolis, Ind.
Empire Mutual Casualty Company, New York, N. Y.
Empire Mutual Insurance Company, Ft. Collins, Colo.
Empire State Mutual Life Insurance Co., Jamestown, N. Y.
Employers Mutual Casualty Co., Des Moines, Iowa
Employers Mutual Insurance Company, Denver, Colo.
Employers Reinsurance Corp., Kansas City, Mo.
Equitable Life Assurance Society of U. S., New York, N. Y.
Equitable National Insurance Co., Des Moines, Iowa
Equity General Insurance Co., Boulder, Colo.
Equity Mutual Insurance Company, Kansas City, Mo.
Erie Indemnity Co., Erie, Pennsylvania
Eureka Casualty Company, Philadelphia, Pa.

Exchange Mutual Indemnity Insurance Co., Buffalo, N. Y.

Factory Mutual Liability Ins. Co. of America, Providence, Rhode Island

Farm Bureau Mutual Insurance Co., Des Moines, Iowa

Farmers American Auto Club, Los Angeles, Calif.

Farmers Casualty Company, Des Moines, Iowa

Farmers Elevator Mutual Casualty Co., Des Moines, Iowa

Farmers Insurance Exchange, Los Angeles, Calif.

Farmers Insurance Group, Los Angeles, Calif.

Farmers Mutual Auto Insurance Co., Madison, Wis.

Farmers New World Life Insurance Co., Los Angeles, Calif.

Federal Insurance Company, New York, N. Y.

Federal Life & Casualty Co., Battle Creek, Mich.

Federal Mutual Casualty Co., Milwaukee, Wis.

Federal Mutual Liability Insurance Co., Boston, Mass.

Federal Surety Company, Davenport, Iowa

Federated Security Insurance Co., Salt Lake City, Utah

Fidelity & Casualty Company, Dallas, Texas

Fidelity & Casualty Co. of New York, New York, N.Y.

Fidelity & Deposit Co. of Maryland, Baltimore, Md.

Fidelity Health & Accident Co., Benton Harbor, Mich.

Fidelity Health Association, Vancouver, B. C., Canada

Fidelity Interstate Life Insurance Co., Philadelphia, Pa.

Fireman's Fund Indemnity Co., San Francisco, Calif. and New York, N. Y.

Firemen's Insurance Company of Newark, Newark, N. J.

First United Life Insurance Company, Gary, Ind.

Fort Wayne Mercantile Accident Ass'n, Fort Wayne, Ind.

Founders Mutual Casualty Company, Chicago, Ill.

Frankenmuth Mutual Auto Insurance Company, Frankenmuth, Mich.

Freeport Insurance Company, Freeport, Ill.

General Accident, Fire & Life Assurance Corp., Ltd., Perth, Scotland, and Philadelphia, Pa.

General Accident Insurance Co., Philadelphia, Pa.
General American Life Insurance Co., St. Louis, Mo.
General Casualty Company, Madison, Wisconsin
General Casualty Company of America, Seattle, Wash.
General Indemnity Exchange, St. Louis, Mo.
George Rogers Clark Casualty Co., Rockford, Ill.
George Washington Insurance Co., Des Moines, Iowa
Georgia Casualty & Surety Co., Atlanta, Ga.
German-Austrian Benevolent Ass'n, St. Louis, Mo.
Glens Falls Insurance Co., Glens Falls, N. Y.
Globe Indemnity Company, New York, N. Y.
Goodville Mutual Casualty Company, Goodville, Pa.
Gopher Mutual Casualty Company, Duluth, Minn.
Government Employees Insurance Co., Washington, D. C.
Grain Dealers Mutual Fire Insurance Company,
    Indianapolis, Ind.
Great American Indemnity Co., New York, N. Y.
Great Eastern Mutual Life Insurance Co., Denver, Colo.
Great Lakes Casualty Company, Detroit, Mich.
Great National Life Ins. Co., Dallas, Texas
Greek Catholic Union of Russian Brotherhoods of USA,
    Munhall, Pennsylvania
Group Health, St. Paul, Minn.
Guarantee Indemnity Company, Indianapolis, Ind.
Guarantee Insurance Company, Los Angeles, Calif.
Guardian Life Insurance Co. of America, New York, N.Y.
Hardware Dealers Mutual Fire Insurance Company,
    Stevens Point, Wis.
Hardware Indemnity Insurance Co. of Minn.,
    Minneapolis, Minn.
Hardware Mutual Casualty Co., Stevens Point, Wis.
Harleysville Mutual Casualty Co., Harleysville, Pa.
Hartford Accident Indemnity Co., Hartford, Conn.
Hartford Steam Boiler Inspection & Insurance Company,
    Hartford, Connecticut
Hawkeye Security Insurance Company, Des Moines, Iowa

Hearthstone Ins. Co. of Massachusetts, Boston, Mass.
Highway Casualty Company, Chicago, Illinois
Home Accident & Health Ins. Co., South Bend, Ind.
Home Indemnity Company, New York, N. Y.
Home Life Insurance Company, New York, N. Y.
Home Mutual Insurance Company, Appleton, Wis.
Home Security Life Insurance Co., Durham, N. C.
Homesteaders Life Co., Des Moines, Iowa
Hoosier Casualty Company, Indianapolis, Ind.
Hudson Mohawk Mutual Insurance Co., Albany, N. Y.
Illinois Commercial Men's Association, Chicago, Ill.
Illinois Commercial News Association, Chicago, Ill.
Illinois Traveling Men's Health Ass'n, Chicago, Ill.
Imperial Life Insurance Company, Asheville, N. C.
Income Guaranty Company, South Bend, Ind.
Indemnity Insurance Company of North America,
      Philadelphia, Pennsylvania
Independence Life & Accident Insurance Co., Louisville,
      Ky.
Independent Order of Odd Fellows, U.S.A.
Indianapolis Life Insurance Co., Indianapolis, Ind.
Industrial Indemnity Company, San Francisco, Calif.
Inland Mutual Insurance Co., Huntington, W. Va.
Insurance Co. of Oregon, Portland, Ore.
Interboro Mutual Indemnity Co., New York, N.Y.
Intercoast Mutual Life Insurance Co., Sacramento, Calif.
Inter-Ocean Insurance Company, Cincinnati, Ohio
Iowa High School Insurance Company, Boone, Iowa
Iowa Mutual Insurance Co., DeWitt, Iowa
Iowa National Mutual Insurance Co., Cedar Rapids, Iowa
Iowa State Traveling Men's Ass'n., Des Moines, Iowa
Jefferson National Life Ins. Co., Indianapolis, Ind.
John Hancock Mutual Life Insurance Co., Boston, Mass.
Kansas City Casualty Company, Denver, Colo.
Kentucky Central Life & Accident Insurance Co.,
      Anchorage, Ky.

Keystone Auto Club Casualty Co., Philadelphia, Pa.
Knights of Pythias, U.S.A.
Kralee Insurance Service, Chicago, Ill.
Lansing Employers Underwriters, Lansing, Mich.
Lawyers Surety Corporation, Dallas, Texas
Liberty Lloyds, Forth Worth, Texas
Liberty Mutual Insurance Co., Boston, Mass.
Life & Casualty Insurance Co. of Tennessee,
    Nashville, Tenn.
Life Insurance Co. of America, Wilmington, Dela.
Life Insurance Company of Georgia, Atlanta, Ga.
Life Insurance Company of the South, Charlotte, N. C.
Lincoln Income Life Insurance Co., Louisville, Ky.
Lincoln Life Insurance Co., Augusta, Ga.
Lincoln Mutual Casualty Company, Detroit, Mich.
Lincoln National Life Insurance Co., Ft. Wayne, Ind.
Lloyds Guarantee Assurance Company, Dallas, Texas
Locomotive Engineers Mutual Life & Accident Ins.
    Assoc., Cleveland, O.
London & Lancashire Indemnity Co. of America,
    Hartford, Connecticut
London Guarantee & Accident Co., Ltd., New York
    and London, England
London Life Insurance Company, London, Ont., Can.
Loyal Protective Life Insurance Co., Boston, Mass.
Lumberman's Mutual Casualty Company, Chicago, Ill.
Madison Co., Mutual Auto Ins. Co., Edwardsville, Ill.
Maine Bonding & Casualty Company, Portland, Me.
Manufacturers Casualty Ins. Co., Philadelphia, Pa.
Manufacturers Liability Ins. Co., Jersey City, N.J.
Maryland Casualty Company, Baltimore, Md.
Masonic Protective Association, Worcester, Mass.
Massachusetts Bonding & Ins. Co., Boston, Mass.
Massachusetts Casualty Insurance Co., Boston, Mass.
Massachusetts Indemnity & Life Insurance Co.,
    Boston, Mass.

Massachusetts Mutual Life Insurance Co.,
    Springfield, Mass.
Massachusetts Protective Ass'n, Inc., Worcester, Mass.
Merchants Casualty Company, Winnipeg, Canada
Merchants Life & Casualty Co., Minneapolis, Minn.
Merchants Mutual Casualty Company, Buffalo, N. Y.
Metals Mutual Insurance Co., Grand Rapids, Mich.
Metropolitan Casualty Insurance Company of New York,
    Newark, N. J.
Metropolitan Life Insurance Co., New York, N. Y.
Michigan Casualty Company, Detroit, Mich.
Michigan Hospital Benefit Association, Detroit, Mich.
Michigan Life Insurance Company, Detroit, Mich.
Michigan Mutual Automobile Insurance Co., Traverse
    City, Michigan
Michigan Mutual Liability Co., Detroit, Mich.
Michigan Surety Company, Lansing, Mich.
Mid-America Insurance Company, Detroit, Mich.
Mid-Century Insurance Company, Los Angeles, Calif.
Midland National Life Ins. Co., Watertown, S. D.
Midwest Life Insurance Co., Lincoln, Nebr.
Midwest Mutual Insurance Co., Des Moines, Iowa
Milwaukee Insurance Company of Milwaukee,
    Milwaukee, Wis.
Ministers Life and Casualty Union, Minneapolis, Minn.
Minnesota Farmers Mutual Casualty Ins. Company,
    Minneapolis, Minn.
Missouri Casualty Company, Clayton, Mo.
Modern Romans, Manistee, Mich.
Modern Woodmen of America, Rock Island, Ill.
Monarch Life Insurance Company, Springfield, Mass.
Motor Club of America Life Insurance Co., Newark, N. J.
Motorist's Protective Association, New York, N. Y.
Mountain States Mutual Ins. Co., Albuquerque, N. M.
Mutual Benefit Life Insurance Co., Newark, N. J.
Mutual Benefit Society of Baltimore City, Baltimore, Md.

Appendix C

Mutual Life Insurance Co. of N. Y., New York, New York
Mutual Protective Insurance Co., Kansas City, Mo.
Mutual Protective Insurance Co., Omaha, Nebr.
Mutual Savings Life Ins. Co., St. Louis, Mo.
National Accident & Health Insurance Co., Philadelphia, Pa.
National Accident Insurance Company, Lincoln, Nebr.
National Auto & Casualty Co., Los Angeles, Calif.
National Ben Franklin Insurance Company of Pittsburgh, Pittsburgh, Pa.
National Casualty Company, Detroit, Mich.
National Casualty Company, Indianapolis, Ind.
National Home Assurance Co., St. Louis, Mo.
National Indemnity Exchange, St. Louis, Mo.
National Life Benefit Co., Houston, Texas
National Life & Casualty Co., Phoenix, Arizona
National Lloyds, Baltimore, Md.
National Masonic Provident Ass'n, Mansfield, Ohio
National Mutual Casualty Co., Detroit, Mich.
National Public Service Insurance Co., Seattle, Wash.
National Sick Benefits Association, Washington, D. C.
National Travelers Benefit Ass'n, Des Moines, Iowa
National Travelers Life Co., Des Moines, Iowa
Nationwide Life Insurance Co., Columbus, Ohio
Nationwide Mutual Insurance Co., Columbus, Ohio
New Amsterdam Casualty Co., Baltimore, Md.
Newark Insurance Co., New York, N. Y.
New England Casualty Company, Boston, Mass.
New England Insurance Co., Springfield, Mass.
New England Mutual Life Ins. Co., Boston, Mass.
New Jersey Manufacturers Casualty Ins. Co., Trenton, N. J.
New York Life Insurance Co., New York, N. Y.
New York Printers & Book Binders Mutual Ins. Co., New York, New York
Norodna Hrvatske Zajednica, Pittsburgh, Pa.

North America Assurance Society of Virginia, Inc.,
  Richmond, Va.
North American Accident Ins. Co., Chicago, Ill.
North American Life and Casualty Company,
  Minneapolis, Minn.
North American Life Ins. Co. of Chicago, Chicago, Ill.
North American Union Life Assurance Society, Chicago,
  Ill.
North Carolina Mutual, Durham, N. C.
North Central Life Insurance Co., St. Paul, Minn.
Northern Casualty Co., Des Moines, Iowa
Northern Life Insurance Co., Seattle, Wash.
Northwestern Life Ins. Co., Seattle, Wash.
Norwich Union Indemnity Co., New York, N. Y.
Occidental Life Ins. Co. of California, Los Angeles, Calif.
Ocean Accident & Guarantee Corp., Ltd., New York,
  N. Y.
Oglethorpe Life Insurance Co., Savannah, Ga.
Ohio Casualty Insurance Co., Hamilton, Ohio
Ohio Farmers Indemnity Co., LeRoy, Ohio
Ohio Farmers Insurance Company, LeRoy, Ohio
Ohio State Life Insurance Co., Columbus, Ohio
Old American Ins. Company, Kansas City, Mo.
Old Colony Insurance Co., Boston, Mass.
Old Line Accident Insurance Co., Lincoln, Nebr.
Old Republic Insurance Co., Chicago, Ill.
Order of Railway Conductors, Cedar Rapids, Iowa
Order of Railway Employees, San Francisco, Calif.
Order of Red Men, Georgetown, Ill.
Order of United Commercial Travelers of America,
  Columbus, Ohio
Pacific Automobile Ins. Co., Los Angeles, Calif.
Pacific Employers Insurance Co., Los Angeles, Calif.
Pacific Indemnity Co., Los Angeles, Calif.
Pacific Mutual Life Ins. Co., Los Angeles, Calif.

Pacific National Fire Insurance Company,
 San Francisco, Calif.
Palatine Insurance Co., New York, N. Y.
Palmetto State Life Ins. Co., Columbia, S. C.
Paul Revere Life Insurance Company, Worcester, Mass.
Peninsular Life Insurance Co., Jacksonville, Fla.
Penn Mutual Life Ins. Co., Philadelphia, Pa.
Pennsylvania Casualty Co., Lancaster, Pa.
Pennsylvania Mfrs. Ass'n Casualty Ins. Company,
 Philadelphia, Pa.
Pa. Threshermen's & Farmers Mutual Cas. Ins. Co.,
 Harrisburg, Pa.
People's Mutual Life Ins. Co., San Francisco, Calif.
Personal Indemnity Co., Milwaukee, Wis.
Phoenix Assurance Co. of New York, New York, N. Y.
Phoenix London Group, Pittsburgh, Pa.
Phoenix Mutual Life Ins. Co., Hartford, Conn.
Pilot Life Insurance Co., Greensboro, N. C.
Pioneer Mutual Casualty Company, Columbus, Ohio
Policyholders Mutual Casualty Co., Des Moines, Iowa
Policyholders National Life Insurance Co., Sioux Falls,
 S. D.
Postal Life & Casualty Co., Kansas City, Mo.
Poulsen Insurance Co. of America, Chicago, Ill.
Preferred Automobile Ins. Co., Grand Rapids, Mich.
Preferred Risk Automobile Insurance Co., Newark, N. J.
Preferred Risk Mutual Insurance Co., Des Moines, Iowa
Progressive Life Insurance Co., Red Bank, N. J.
Progressive Mutual Ins. Co., Cleveland, Ohio
Protective Association of Canada, Granby, Quebec,
 Canada
Providence Washington Insurance Co., Providence, R. I.
Provident Accident & White Cross Ins. Co., Ltd.,
 New York, N. Y.
Provident Indemnity Life Ins. Co., Norristown, Pa.
Prudential Life Ins. Co. of America, Newark, N. J.

Public Mutual Casualty Co., St. Louis, Mo.
Pullman Company, United States of America
Queen Insurance Company, New York, N. Y.
Reliable Life Insurance Co., Webster Grove, Mo.
Reliance Insurance Co., Philadelphia, Pa.
Reliance Life Insurance Co. of Georgia, Atlanta, Ga.
Reliance Mutual Life Ins. Co., Park Ridge, Ill.
Republic Indemnity Co., Columbus, Ohio
Reserve National Insurance Co., Oklahoma City, Okla.
Rhode Island Mutual Ins. Co., Providence, R. I.
Ridgeley Protective Association, Worcester, Mass.
Rockford Life Insurance Co., Rockford, Ill.
Royal General Insurance Company of Canada
Royal-Globe Insurance Group, New York, N. Y.
Royal Indemnity Co., New York, N. Y.
Safeguard Insurance Company, Hartford, Conn.
Safety Casualty Co., Dallas, Texas
St. Paul-Mercury Indemnity Co. of St. Paul, Minn.
Secured Insurance Company, Indianapolis 6, Indiana
Security Life & Trust Co., Winston-Salem, N. C.
Security Mutual Casualty Co., Chicago, Ill.
Security Mutual Life Ins. Co., Binghamton, N. Y.
Security Mutual Life Insurance Co., Lincoln, Nebr.
Selected Risks Indemnity Co., Branchville, N. J.
Service Casualty Co., New York, N. Y.
Service Mutual Insurance Co. of Texas
Skyland Life Insurance Co., Charlotte, N. C.
Societee Des Artisans Insurance Co., Montreal, Que.
S. D. Employers Protective Ass'n, Sioux Falls, S. D.
Southern Casualty Co., Alexandria, Louisiana
Southern Life Insurance Co., Baltimore, Md.
Southern National Insurance Co., Little Rock, Ark.
Southern Surety Co., Des Moines, Iowa
Southland Life Insurance Co., Dallas, Texas
Standard Accident Insurance Co., Detroit, Mich.
Standard Life Assn., Lawrence, Kansas

248

Standard Life & Casualty Insurance Co., Rock Hill, S. C.
Star Insurance Co. of America, New York; N. Y.
State Auto Insurance Ass'n, Des Moines, Iowa
State Automobile Mutual Insurance Co. of Ohio
State Capitol (Life) Insurance Co., Raleigh, N. C.
State Compensation Ins. Fund, San Francisco, Calif.
State Farm Mutual Automobile Insurance Company,
     Bloomington, Illinois
State Insurance Co. of Kentucky, Louisville, Ky.
State Life Insurance Co. of Colorado, Denver, Colo.
State Mutual Benefit Society, Philadelphia, Pa.
State Mutual Life Assurance Co. of America,
     Worcester, Mass.
Stuyvesant Life Insurance Co., Allentown, Pa.
Suburban Casualty Co., Wheaton, Ill.
Sun Indemnity Company of New York, New York, N.Y.
Sun Insurance Co. of New York, New York, N. Y.
Sun Life Insurance Co., Los Angeles, Calif.
Sunset Life Insurance Co. of America, Olympia, Wash.
Superior Lloyds of America, Dallas, Texas
Supreme Casualty Co., Milwaukee, Wis.
Teachers Prot. Mutual Life Ins. Co., Lancaster, Pa.
Texas Employers Insurance Co., Dallas, Texas
Textile Insurance Co., High Point, N. C.
The Continental Insurance Company, New York, N. Y.
The Crown Life Insurance Co., Toronto, Canada
The Employers Liability Assurance Corp., Ltd.,
     Boston, Mass.
The Gem City Life Insurance Co., Dayton, Ohio
The Halifax Insurance Company of Mass., Boston, Mass.
The Maccabees, Detroit, Mich.
The State Hospital Assoc., Inc., Tarboro, N.C.
Threshermen's Mutual Ins. Co., Fond du Lac, Wis.
Time Insurance Co., Milwaukee, Wis.
Title Guaranty & Casualty Co. of America, Detroit, Mich.
Transit Casualty Co., St. Louis, Mo.

Transit Mutual Insurance Co., Boston, Mass.
Transport Indemnity Co., Los Angeles, Calif.
Transportation Insurance Co., Chicago, Ill.
Transportation Mutual Ins. Co., Boston, Mass.
Travelers Indemnity Co., Hartford, Conn.
Travelers Insurance Co., Hartford, Conn.
Travelers Protective Ass'n of America, St. Louis, Mo.
Travelers Protective Ass'n, Kokomo, Ind.
Tri-State Insurance Co., Tulsa, Okla.
Truck Insurance Exchange, Los Angeles, Calif.
Twentieth Century Mutual Ins. Co., Detroit, Mich.
Underwriters at Lloyds, London, Frankfort, Ky.
Union Assurance Society, New York, N. Y.
Union Mutual Life Insurance Company, Portland, Maine
United Ass'n of Journeymen Plumbers & Steamfitters,
    U. S. and Canada
United Casualty Co., Westfield, Mass.
United Central Life Ins. Co., Ft. Wayne, Ind.
United Commercial Travelers Ass'n, Utica, N. Y.
United Mine Workers of America, U. S. A.
United Pacific Insurance Co., Tacoma, Wash.
United States Casualty Co., New York, N. Y.
United States Fidelity & Guaranty Co., Baltimore, Md.
United States Guarantee Co., New York, N. Y.
U. S. Government Employees Insurance Co., Wash.,
    D. C.
U. S. Letter Carriers Ass'n, Lancaster, Pa .
U. S. Life Insurance Co. of New York, New York, N. Y.
U. S. Mutual Liability Ins. Co., Quincy, Mass.
Universal Underwriters Insurance Company,
    Kansas City, Mo.
University Life Insurance Co., Indianapolis, Ind.
Utilities Insurance Co., St. Louis, Mo.
Vermont Accident Insurance Co., Rutland, Vt.
Virginia Health & Accident Ass'n, Richmond, Va.
Virginia Mutual Ins. Co., Richmond, Va.

War Risk Insurance Bureau of the Treasury Dept.,
  Washington, D. C.

Washington National Insurance Co., Evanston, Ill.

Western Casualty & Surety Co., Fort Scott, Kansas

Western Reserve Mutual Casualty Co., Wooster, Ohio

Western States Mutual Auto Ins. Co., Freeport, Ill.

Western Surety Co., Sioux Falls, S. D.

Western Travelers Accident Ass'n of California,
  Los Angeles, Calif.

White Cross Plan of the Bankers Life and Casualty
  Company of Chicago, Illinois

Wisconsin Casualty Co., Green Bay, Wis.

Wisconsin National Life Insurance Co., Oshkosh, Wis.

Wolverine Insurance Co., Battle Creek, Mich.

Wolverine Mutual Ins. Co., Dowagiac, Mich.

Woodmen Accident & Life Company, Lincoln, Nebr.

Woodmen Circle, Supreme Forest, Omaha, Nebr.

World Marine General Insurance Company (Canada)

World Mutual Health & Accident Co. of Pennsylvania,
  Philadelphia, Pa.

Wright Mutual Insurance Co., Detroit, Mich.

Zurich Insurance Company, Chicago, Ill.

APPENDIX D

Chiropractic Colleges in the United States and Canada

The major professional organizations of chiropractic in the United States, Canada, and Europe are:

National Chiropractic Association
National Building
Webster City, Iowa

International Chiropractors Association
838 Brady Street
Davenport, Iowa

Canadian Chiropractic Association
252 Bloor Street, West
Toronto, Canada

European Chiropractic Union—Belgium
5 Rue de la Limite
Brussels, Belgium

European Chiropractic Union—Switzerland
44 Blvd. des Tranchees
Geneva, Switzerland

Students who wish to prepare themselves for entrance into the chiropractic profession may obtain full information by contacting these professional associations or the State Board of Chiropractic Examiners in the state in which they wish to practice.

Atlantic States Chiropractic Institute △
555 Fifth Avenue
Brooklyn 15, New York

Canadian Memorial Chiropractic College ○
252 Bloor Street, West
Toronto, Ontario, Canada

Chiropractic Institute of New York ○
325 East 38th Street
New York 16, New York

Cleveland Chiropractic College of Kansas City △
3724 Troost Avenue
Kansas City, Missouri

Cleveland Chiropractic College of Los Angeles △
3511 West Olympic Boulevard
Los Angeles, California

Columbia Institute of Chiropractic △
261 West 71st Street
New York, New York

International Chiropractic College △
1901 E. 5th Street
Dayton 3, Ohio

Lincoln Chiropractic College ○
633 N. Pennsylvania Street
Indianapolis 4, Indiana

Logan Basic College of Chiropractic △
7701 Florissant Road
St. Louis, Missouri

Los Angeles College of Chiropractic O
920 East Broadway
Glendale 5, California

National College of Chiropractic O
20 N. Ashland Boulevard
Chicago 7, Illinois

Northwestern College of Chiropractic O
2222 Park Avenue
Minneapolis, Minnesota

Palmer College of Chiropractic △
1000 Brady Street
Davenport, Iowa

Texas Chiropractic College O
San Pedro Park
San Antonio, Texas

Western States Chiropractic College O
4525 S.E. 63rd Avenue
Portland, Oregon

O—accredited by N.C.A.
△—accredited by I.C.A.

"The doctor of the future will give no medicine, but will interest his patients in the care of the human frame, in diet, and in the cause and prevention of disease."

— THOMAS ALVA EDISON